C000181863

Kick Start Fat Loss The Revolution

The smart woman's guide to losing fat, feeling sharp and transforming health.

by Rachel Holmes

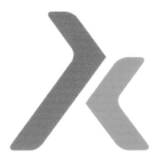

ISBN 978-0-9935416-0-5

Published by Rachel Holmes.
For more copies of this book, please
email: Lesley@Choreographytogo.com
Tel: 07854 739285

Although every precaution has been taken in the preparation of this book, the publisher and author assume no responsibility for errors or omissions. Neither is any liability assumed for damages resulting from the use of this information contained herein.

Kick Start Fat Loss The Revolution

Preface

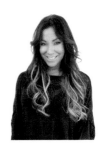

It's a month before Christmas and I'm putting the last few pages together for this book.

I began writing *Kick Start Fat Loss The Revolution* book two years ago which in the nutrition and fitness industry is a lifetime.

It's a fast paced industry with new information and updates coming out all the time.

And, with over 27 years being immersed in it, still my own knowledge and experience grow on a daily basis.

As pioneering research is published and new techniques are discovered I enthusiastically apply it to my own regime, with my personal clients and international *Kick Start Fat Loss* groups.

My ultimate goal is to help millions of women get the best possible results physically and mentally through cutting edge nutrition and fitness.

I'm challenging myths and misconceptions, smashing old hand me down weight loss theories that are totally outdated and ineffective and empowering YOU to become an informed consumer.

Kick Start Fat Loss has become so much more than dropping a dress size or losing a few stone(s) in weight, it's become a movement, a lifestyle ...

... a revolution?

Taking your health into your own hands is crucial to living and loving a happy, healthy, productive life free from minor health niggles, stress, disease, weight gain and body confidence issues.

The first step is understanding nutrition. Becoming a diet detective.

Understanding why and how the food we eat affects EVERYTHING.

Not only how we look but how we feel, how we think, our emotions, our mood, our energy and ultimately our happiness.

Getting your health and nutrition information off the back of a cereal box is going to lock you down into dieting hell for life.

It's not a happy place to be.

I hope this book will challenge your dieting and weight loss beliefs.

I want to encourage you to think deeper about your food choices and gain a thirst for more knowledge.

At first *Kick Start Fat Loss* might seem like a huge mountain to climb.

There's a lot of information here.

It can seem scary. Daunting even. There is so much information that will seem to conflict with what you read in popular magazines or see in the national press - with what's on TV or endorsed by celebrities.

That information is so deeply ingrained into the brain and society that we rarely question it.

Even though it clearly doesn't work long term.

We get stuck into a pattern of thinking it's lack of will power, or we aren't being strict enough, or we just need to find the right plan for now.

And so it continues. On and on ...

So, throughout the book I have popped in many of our *Kick Start Fat Loss* success stories.

Women who have tried everything, were at their wits end, feeling crap, unhappy and not able to understand what was so wrong with their dieting.

These stories are so inspirational.

They became unchained from food, jumped of the dieting roller coaster and embraced a healthy lifestyle.

The *Kick Start Fat Loss* Revolution is dedicated to smart women searching for a life free from short term dieting fixes. It's about women making smart food choices and understanding why some foods make you thrive whilst others stop you dead in your tracks.

It's about choosing the best and most effective exercise and workouts for you.

It's all here!

This is just the first step on an exciting journey.

Let's do this!

Tweet #KSFLREV

Acknowledgements

Thank you: Jayne Nicholls who has been a constant support, motivator and inspiration in all things fitness, business and life related; Val and John for never ending advice; Karen Lisa Laing for awesome writing, editing and finally bringing this project to life; Lesley for dealing with everything I throw at her so patiently; Lauren for aiding and abetting my crazy project ideas; My top girls - Keeley, Terri, Nikki, Gillian, Kelly Reed-Banks, Lisa B, Lisa C - love you ladies; All the fantastic *Kick Start Fat Loss* Franchisees who are doing a smashing job helping so many people look and feel their absolute best.

It's only the beginning.

Introduction

Would you like to know how you could lose weight, feel more energised and stay in shape for life without ever counting a calorie?

Would you like to know how you could balance your hormones and understand what food does to your body?

Would you like to know why cutting calories might be harmful to your weight loss efforts long term and could actually be trapping you in a dieting cycle?

I'm Rachel Holmes, creator of *Kick Start Fat Loss* and I believe I have a lot of information about dieting, exercise, hormones and fat that might just help you out.

Thousands of people across the UK, Ireland and Europe who are already on the *Kick Start Fat Loss* programme have lost pound after pound of fat and have seen inches disappear. Many of these people are women who had tried every diet going until they finally lost those stubborn pounds (or stones) by making some simple but really clever changes to their lifestyle.

Throughout this book you'll be hearing from those people. Real people who have finally found the secret to losing weight and feeling great, for good.

The diet trap

So welcome wonderful lady. Thank you for joining me.

I know you've been at this place before. Starting out on a new diet, except this time you are really going to do it.

There's the initial excitement and resolve. Then the first few days of blissful 'treats' denial, which often involves sharing your smug new dieting status with the world: "No, I'm sorry, I can't have that. I'm on a diet!"

Let's admit it, it's sort of exciting starting a new diet. Especially when it's the one that everyone's talking about and that's a bit, 'out there.'

It works for a bit, maybe even for a bit more. You lose a few pounds or even a stone and squeeze into a new slimline frock. But then comes a party, Christmas, holidays or the friends you've been dieting with slowly start to cave in to temptation and gradually the pounds creep back on.

Would you like to know why that happens?

Calorie counting is not the answer
What would you say if I told you that calorie counting is not the answer? The world didn't even know what a calorie was until the 19th century and there was no obesity epidemic.

Are you addicted to the diet industry?

Have you considered that your food choices might be the result of an addiction, not a lack of willpower? Or that your normal brain function might have been affected by the 'diet foods' that are supposed to make us thin?

And what of the dieting industry - that multi-million dollar industry? Back in 2002 the Federal Trade Commission released a report which estimated as much as 55% of advertising for weight loss products and services contained claims which were false or lacked evidence (Cleland, 2002)[1] The findings sparked a committee aimed at protecting consumers by introducing guidelines but the diet industry along with the fitness industry is self regulated. There are no compulsory codes of conduct.

Even the leading players in the dieting industry have been implicated as having made false claims. In 2010, two of the world's biggest weight loss companies went head to head when Jenny Craig claimed its clients lost over twice as much weight as the leading weight loss company, implicating Weight Watchers (with more than 43% market share in the US). Weight Watchers in turn stated that no clinical trials had been carried out to prove this statement and therefore these claims were misleading. The two companies reached a settlement but those clinical trials have still never been undertaken.

If you got a manicure which didn't last, you would probably choose a different nail technician next time. If your child learned nothing and didn't progress after a term at school you would be asking some serious questions. So why is it that we try the same diet time after time and don't consider something new? What factors are consistently making you fail?

The average woman has been on 61 diets
According to a 2012 survey, the average woman has been on 61 diets by the time she's 45. The poll, undertaken by Warburtons Bakery (HOVIS), found that out of the 2000 women surveyed, the average diet lasted just 15 days and 35% of women put more weight back on after the diet than they'd lost in the first place.

Does this sound familiar? If it does, then you're in the right place. I'd like to help you break your cycle of dieting for good.

The key to losing weight starts with regulating your hormones. Especially your blood sugar and your cortisol levels. This is the starting point for the *Kick Start Fat Loss* detox. I'll show you how to do this.

I'm also going to share with you a lot of information on how your body works and how it processes foods, so you can understand why certain foods or activities may not be helping your efforts for a leaner body.

I'm going to encourage you to become your own diet detective, seeking out the foods that will serve you and those that won't.

I'm going to share a lot of evidence, science and research on exactly why some popular diets or health myths are just not good for you.

---

[1] Cleland, R. (2002), *Weight Loss Advertising: An Analysis of Current Trends*, US:DIANE publishing

I'm also going to share a lot of evidence, science and research on what could work for you. The same information that's helped an army of *Kick Start Fat Loss* recruits achieve their dream weight and inch loss goals - and to feel so much better.

The *Kick Start Fat Loss* Army

I can't prove this works alone. That would be a pretty rubbish survey of 1. I've got help from my growing army of *Kick Start Fat Loss* participants across the UK and Ireland who have dropped a serious amount of fat and literally changed their lives by having faith in *Kick Start Fat Loss*.

A theory with no evidence isn't going to get far in life and I know that there are always arguments for and against but you can't argue with what has worked and is working for my amazing *Kick Start Fat Loss* team.

So I asked a few of the many amazing women who have achieved incredible results to share how and why they finally did it and what was so different. These are all women, real women, probably like you, who have tried lots of diets but never succeeded or maintained their success.

Lesley Gooch

Lesley started *Kick Start Fat Loss* at Fen Park Primary School at the end of June 2013. Lesley is by far one of *Kick Start Fat Loss*'s biggest success stories. She has completely transformed her life and lost over nine stone in the process. Lesley recently travelled with me to Ireland when we took *Kick Start Fat Loss* over there. She was and is a super star. Lesley is 47 and lives in Lowestoft. Here is her *Kick Start Fat Loss* story:

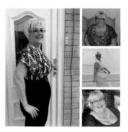

> *Before starting Kick Start Fat Loss I had probably tried every diet going, from Slimming World, Atkins, Weight Watchers and Slim fast to just counting calories. I thought that the most important things I had to do to lose weight were to count calories, eat smaller portions and stick to low fat food. I'd lost a stone here and there but soon put it and more back on. I was fed up of trying every diet going only to put weight back on.*

> *I was making myself ill with the amount of weight I was carrying around. Plus it was getting embarrassing working in a school and sitting on little chairs.*

> *I found out about Kick Start Fat Loss through Helen, my Kick Start Fat Loss instructor. We'd originally met when I'd attended her circuit training classes but it was only when she friended me on Facebook that I found out about Kick Start Fat Loss. I was impressed by how much weight and how many inches Helen's clients had lost. So when she said Rachel was coming to Lowestoft I thought I would check it out.*

> *I thought it might be the same as all the other diets but Helen's clients had such good weight and inch loss results in such a short time, so I thought if I could achieve the same I wouldn't get fed up with it so easily.*

> *Rachel explained how the diet worked and about giving up sugar and processed foods, so I thought it would be worth trying especially since exercise was included in the plan.*

> *Kick Start Fat Loss was so easy to follow and I lost 15 pounds in the first week. Since I started, ten months ago, I have lost weight every week except one.*

> *At first I was nervous of the exercise part of it because I was so fat. I thought people would think, 'why is she doing this,' or 'she is too fat to manage this.' On other diets I'd joined the gym but felt very embarrassed to go on any of the equipment so I just did swimming. But the girls were so welcoming and helped me to stop feeling embarrassed. Helen and the girls would encourage me along and I soon started to enjoy it. It soon became fun to meet with the girls each week. Although we work very hard we all have a laugh and we all support each other. We all feel so happy when each of us loses the weight and support each other if we have had a bad week.*

> *In the beginning Helen modified some of the exercises for me. I was so fat and unhealthy that couldn't manage much. So I would do step touches instead of jogging,*

knee lifts instead of jumping and power walking instead of running. Helen said as long as my heart rate was up I was burning fat and getting the benefits.

As I gradually lost the weight and became fitter I could manage the original exercises. But there were other benefits too. I've had asthma since I was a child and the more weight I put on the worse it got. I found that I couldn't walk up the stairs without wheezing. When I started Kick Start Fat Loss I found I had to use the inhaler a lot when I was exercising but now, 10 months on, my asthma is better and I maybe only take it once during the workout.

I've made lots of changes for good. I eat healthy foods and have cut out all the rubbish like bread and crisps. I now find I can't eat anything like that, so I am really hopeful this will be a complete lifestyle change, for the rest of my life.

I now exercise three to four times a week and I've bought a bike (I hadn't ridden a bike for around 10 years).

Kick Start Fat Loss was so easy to follow and all the changes make you feel so much healthier and fitter. It's a lifestyle change rather than a diet, more of an easy eating and exercise plan. You eat only healthy foods. No sugar. No low fat products. No own diet club foods.

I am so much fitter now and happier too. I don't feel depressed or grumpy about my weight anymore. I have so much more energy and feel a whole lot better about how I look. And it's easier to sit on the little chairs at school.

Lynette Culverwell

----

22 months ago you would have found an unhappy and unfit 18 stone 7lbs Lynette Culverwell. The 34-year-old mum of one from Lowestoft had spent countless years calorie counting and following low fat diets in an attempt to lose weight. In July 2013 she started *Kick Start Fat Loss* in Lowestoft. Here is Lynette's story:

Whilst attending a *Kick Start Fat Loss* open evening, Lynette was introduced to a completely new way of eating that focused on nutrition rather than obsessive calorie counting. Here is Lynette's *Kick Start Fat Loss* story:

> *Kick Start Fat Loss encourages people to focus on the foods you eat, the source it comes from and the way it makes you feel. It's a complete lifestyle change which works on building healthier relationships with food so that you stop 'dieting' and start living.*

> *Before Kick Start Fat Loss my daily food intake would typically be nothing for breakfast, cheese sandwiches and crisps for lunch and sausage casserole with yorkshire pudding and mash for dinner. Since Joining Kick Start Fat Loss I have learnt to enjoy eating again.*

> *I love cooking all of my meals from scratch knowing I am eating clean, nutritious food. I have a local vegetable box delivered on a Friday and do my grocery shopping on a Saturday based around the contents of my vegetable box. My husband and I both work full-time and bring up our son so life is hectic but Kick Start Fat Loss is just part of it.*

> *Typical meals now include bacon and spinach omelette with a green juice for breakfast, homemade soup for lunch and salmon and steak with vegetables for dinner.*

> *I've said goodbye to emotional eating too. I used to snack daily on chocolate, biscuits and sugar. I loved comfort food. If I was upset about something I would eat large sharing size bars of chocolate and massive bags of crisps to make me feel better. I thought nothing about eating a whole tub of Ben and Jerry's all to myself.*

> *I can now eat guilt free, since I know the food I'm eating is helping me to become slimmer, healthier and stronger.*

> *Before Kick Start Fat Loss, I would have dismissed the idea of joining an exercise. I had low self esteem and felt embarrassed. Kick Start Fat Loss has given me the confidence to exercise. I now train at the gym and take part in exercise classes like Pilates, Boxfit and HIIT.*

> *Family outings used to make me embarrassed because of my size and weight. There was a limit to what I could do. So I would often miss out on the fun and volunteer to stay with the bags and buggy instead. I was petrified of queuing only to get to the front and not be able to fit into the car or harness. I have just returned from Disneyland Paris I can proudly confirm that I went on everything and had no such fears!*

On Valentine's Day 2014 my husband proposed. Four months later we were married. I had lost six stone and felt like a princess. Although my weight loss meant I had to have 11 inches off my wedding dress.

I have now lost an amazing eight stone. I look and feel incredible. I couldn't have done it without Kick Start Fat Loss. I've learned to make the right choices about the foods I eat.

The group offers amazing support and have been like a family to me. I have met some amazing people and made new friendships. Helen Pybus has been an inspirational mentor and my journey wouldn't have been possible without her.

I'm excited about the future and want others to feel as good as I do. Try Kick Start Fat Loss - there is nothing else out there like it. You will be amazed with the results you get. It's given me my life back and I can run around with my son and shop in 'normal' clothes shops. I don't have to pretend to be happy anymore. I am happy.

Rachel and Johnnie Ellis

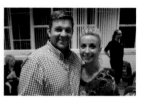

Rachel and Johnnie are a busy couple balancing four children and a stressful job in Thetford, Norfolk. They are a real inspiration. They ditched their old diets and started clean eating with *Kick Start Fat Loss*. They started *Kick Start Fat Loss* with Michelle Jermy in Thetford in July 2015. Here's their story:

My diet on the whole had always been okay - or so I thought. I would eat a bowl of cereal for breakfast, a sandwich and a bag of crisps for lunch. I would snack on fruit during the day and have a meal in the evening, usually a potato or pasta based meal.

I was getting fed up with my constant lack of energy every afternoon. I would feel so sluggish and would use chocolate to get me through. Some days, I felt so exhausted I felt like taking a nap. I had also been experiencing a horrible bloated and cramping feeling in my tummy regularly after meals.

I've always enjoyed exercising and keeping fit and although I'd never attended any slimming clubs in the past, I would try to follow all the advice out there. For years, I'd bought the low fat versions of food believing I was doing myself and my family a favour. I didn't realise we were over-dosing on sugar. If I felt hungry, I'd snack on a bowl of cereal, thinking I was taking the healthy option.

I'm a busy stay-at-home mum with four children aged 21, 19, 15 and 3! Having a baby at the age of 43 was a big deal.

My husband Johnnie has a stressful job, owning and managing a busy manufacturing company. He would start his day with a bowl of cereal and survive the rest of his working day on 10 or 12 cups of coffee and tea, each loaded with two spoonfuls of sugar. With every hot drink he had a couple of biscuits. A recipe for disaster! After his evening meal, he would snack on something sweet - usually chocolate (and I would join him).

Six years previously, Johnnie signed up to the Lighter Life program in a desperate bid to lose weight. This diet consisted of powdered shakes, soups and the occasional snack bar. He lost six stone in a relatively short time but once he started to eat food again, he piled every pound back on – plus quite a few more! It was a miserable time for him.

We were introduced to Kick Start Fat Loss by Michelle Jermy. She is an inspirational lady and an amazing Yoga and Pilates instructor. I had been attending her classes at The Core Studio in my home town of Thetford, Norfolk. Because of her positive outlook and the results I was achieving through attending her classes, I decided that Johnnie could also benefit, so I signed him up to some personal training sessions with her.

Although he was exercising regularly, his weight wasn't easily shifting. His diet needed attention. We are now both in our mid forties and very aware of the fact that our health cannot be taken for granted. We needed help.

Michelle had spoken to us about Kick Start Fat Loss and suggested that we gave it a go - as a family. I was really keen to see if it would make any positive changes to the way I was feeling - and if I could shift the weight I was hanging on to around my middle.
Although I'm not classed as overweight, I'd begun to feel uncomfortable but had been putting it down to 'middle aged spread'. I had almost accepted it was there to stay!

We've now been on the plan for two months and we're loving everything about it. I have lost half a stone - much of that is from my tummy. Johnnie has lost an incredible 19lbs. My bloated tummy cramps have disappeared completely and I'm feeling much more energised. I don't suffer the dreadful drop in energy levels during the afternoons anymore. It's also done wonders for my libido!

I thought the hardest part of this new lifestyle would be cutting out the bread, pasta and potatoes but I've been pleasantly surprised. I don't miss these things at all and feel so much better for cutting them out.

I still have one coffee every day but I've switched to a really nice organic one, which I thoroughly enjoy. I didn't realise the amount of hidden sugar we were consuming in our food. By eliminating it from our diet, it seems our taste buds really appreciate what we do eat now and I'm not craving chocolate like I once was.

For Johnnie, cutting out the caffeine initially created a few problems. He had a week of headaches and felt rough. He was a complete nightmare to live with during that time! It's been more than worth it though - two months on and he doesn't drink tea or coffee at all now.

I've found incorporating Kick Start Fat Loss into our family life easy - although my 15 year old son is still getting used to it. He hasn't been impressed with the lack of chocolate and snacks.

Sticking to it when we're socialising hasn't created the problems I thought it might. Most restaurants now cater for gluten free customers and we often ask to swap potatoes and pasta for extra vegetables. If I'm entertaining at home, I prepare a 'clean' meal as normal and our guests enjoy it.

My best friend in the kitchen nowadays is my spiraliser. It has given my vegetables a new lease of life. I can substitute pasta for some delicious courgetti spaghetti or blitz a cauliflower head to replace rice.

Because we have seen such positive results in all areas of our life, we firmly believe that Kick Start Fat Loss is the way to go and we would recommend it to anyone.

We'd like to thank Michelle for all her nurturing and for introducing us to this lifestyle. From listening to Michelle and Rachel Holmes, we have learnt so much – it all makes perfect sense.

The Woman Power Diet

This book is not just another diet book. I like to think of it more as a bit of girl power - well actually woman power. This woman shares what she knows with lots of other women and helps to make them happier, healthier and thinner.

Kick Start Fat Loss changes lives

Over the past two years I've developed a system which has literally changed lives. *Kick Start Fat Loss* is currently running in over 100 locations around the UK, Ireland and Europe. From Scotland to Gibralter (more on how it came to be later). Each location has between 50 and 2000 participants doing *Kick Start Fat Loss* on a weekly basis.

Across those groups, in the first 28 days participants lose on average 11 and a half pounds and six inches, most of which comes off around the middle. And, 80% of participants stick with the program and go on to get great results.

Yes I know diets sell and instead I'm trying to share with you major lifestyle change. But my 'diet' could not only get you weight loss results, it could give you control over your willpower, mental clarity and increased confidence. They are all part of the package.

My biggest losers and life changers

You've already met superstars Lesley and Lynette but here are a few more:

- Mum of two, Jackie Panks from Norfolk, who lost 26 inches of body fat in 12 months.

- Health care assistant, Victoria Brodie-Smith from North London, who lost three and a half stone on *Kick Start Fat Loss*.

- *Kick Start Fat Loss* West Wickham franchise owner, Chris Tuck, who now manages her eating disorders and mental health through clean eating.

- Mum of five, 40-year-old Kim Lee from Croydon, who lost over six stone and has got medical approval for the breast reduction she's always wanted.

- *Kick Start Fat Loss* instructor, Sindy Matthews, who lost two stone in six months, inspite of already being fit and active.

- Lisa Lockwood from Lowestoft, who went from yo yo dieting to losing over three stone.

- 47-year-old Carlie Goode from Banbury, who is overcoming debilitating M.E. through *Kick Start Fat Loss* eating principles.

Kick Start Fat Loss is based on sound research

Kick Start Fat Loss is about re-educating and debunking nutrition, fat loss and weight loss myths that have become ingrained in our culture and I want to share this research with womankind! I'll tell you a little secret: I'd like to go global! But let's just start with me and you.

I want to share the knowledge. If you buy this book and give it to your friend and it works, FAB! I have little interest in locking you down to buy Rachel's cottage cheese or Rachel's kitchen scales. I want you to stop failing and finally achieve the body you want.

I want you to understand how and why *Kick Start Fat Loss* works
My focus is on education. I want you to understand how and why it works rather than just asking you to believe me.

Before social media, the diet and nutrition news and information that hit the headlines was either sensationalised for a good news story and disseminated through newspapers, magazines or television news, or it came from well established diet companies with big marketing budgets.

The social media diet revolution
The best thing that could have happened for your waistline in recent years is social media. For years, since I discovered the truth about getting in great shape I've felt like a tiny voice in the corner saying, "Please listen to me - I have the truth," but without a multi-million dollar media machine to drive my message forwards I would always be a little voice.

For every sweeping statement about sugar, fructose or fat there is a sound, evidence based argument which I don't believe is getting through and that's where I'm coming from.

I would love for you to finish this book with questions answered and with an understanding of how your body stores fat, reacts to hormones and what are the major factors preventing you from having the body shape or health you are striving after. And if you still have questions at the end of all of this, please ask me.

Who am I?

So why listen to me?

Let's go back a little. I feel like I've been all sales pitch and no introductions.

Whilst I'm not a megalomaniac or a self absorbed wannabe, I'd like you to invest some time and effort in me, therefore I think a little introduction is both polite and important to your understanding of *Kick Start Fat Loss*.

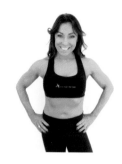

I was born an entrepreneur
I was born and raised in Nottingham, so as you read this I'd like you to add a little northern twang! My mum and dad were publicans so we lived in a pub. They owned the business. My dad is an unbelievable entrepreneur. He always said to me and my brother that we should always work for ourselves. Never work for anyone else. And we've both followed our passions. I suppose you could say I was born an entrepreneur.

The fitness thing all started when I was 14. My brother and me were BMX champions. I was European and British champion and we were looking for something to do in the winter (my brother is still a BMX champion - he lives in the US and has more titles than anyone else in the world).

So we both joined a little spit and sawdust gym in the local town. Ilkestone in Derbyshire.

Love at first grapevine
The gym had an aerobics class. A Jane Fonda style aerobics class. I joined it and it was love at first grapevine. By the time I was 16, I was teaching in that same gym.

I also set up my own classes, in the function room of our pub. It was £2 to come and the first class got around 20 people. And that's how it all started!

At the time there was no governing body for aerobics. When the first qualification came out, from the YMCA, I jumped at it and at nearly 18 I completed the first YMCA Teaching Exercise to Music qualification to run outside of London (I was just old enough to drive to the training venue).

I was doing something different
I was the youngest by far. All the rest were keep fit, popmobility ladies who'd been teaching for years! They were lovely ladies but I was doing something different. I was buying records from the local DJ and mixing up Rick Astley and stuff (I can assure you back then they were pop classics).

It was the late 80s. It was Thatcher. It was girl power. It was Cosmopolitan. It was a very different time, it was a great time to be starting out as an entrepreneur.

Nobody ran their own business
When I left school everybody went to work in a factory, either hosiery or pottery. Nobody worked for themselves. Nobody's parents work for themselves. Nobody ran their own business. So there I was, in the 80s, in the middle of a girl power movement, going against

the grain and being different. It was a good time to get going. In fact it was a great time to be starting a fitness business.

Along came the 90s. Freestyle fitness was in its heyday and throughout the next few decades gyms and health clubs grew in popularity and fitness became big business. My business grew with it.

I knew that most diets didn't work

From conventions to fitness events, I was there presenting. I loved it. I had my business Choreography to Go and I knew all the big names in fitness. I had my name to aerobics music compilations, I worked with Kelly Holmes and Mel B, I was sponsored by Nike and Red Bull. I was a pretty major player. And because I was always in the thick of it I also knew the ins and outs of the dieting industry. How diets and fitness were being sold to the average person (usually women) and I knew that most diets didn't work.

My main market was the fitness professional rather than the (and excuse the expression) 'end user' - the punter! I'd built my business before the advent of social media. I could keep in touch with fitness professionals but to grow to the size of the punter meant big budgets that I didn't have. So until a few years ago all was good in Miss Rachel's business world. I was an independent woman, doing what I loved and pretty comfortable thank you very much.

Emergency surgery

Then everything changed. I went from invincible Miss Rachel, to surgery to save my sight in what seemed like the blink of an eye. What started as a routine trip to the doctors for a headache, had me in emergency surgery for a detached retina in less than 24 hours.

Inspired by my life shock, I designed *Kick Start Fat Loss*

I was at risk of not being able to see again, let alone work, drive or be independent. Inspired by my life shock, I designed *Kick Start Fat Loss*. And during my six week recuperation I built it!

The threat to my sight spurred me into action. I used the contacts I'd built up and the industry knowledge I had. I'd always wanted to get a true, honest diet and fitness programme out there to rival those I knew about which didn't give the full picture and with the advent of social media I could suddenly do it.

Kick Start Fat Loss is about getting fit for good

I was sick of hearing about calorie controlled diets. I was fed up of hearing the dieting woes of these poor women who were in a dieting yo-yo cycle. They lost the weight, the weight came back on and over time it got harder to drop the weight in the first place. Not only that but these women were not looking after themselves. They were getting sick. And they were starving hungry and grumpy with dieting!

This is where *Kick Start Fat Loss* is different. It's about fat but it's also about health. It's about changing unhealthy eating habits. It's about getting fit for good.

What I love about it, is that it uses the team of fitness professionals I've built up over the years and helps them build a business and a community too. I'm not in this to make wads of cash. As I've said, I was doing fine as an independent business woman and still am. *Kick Start Fat Loss* is more than a business venture for me. Without wishing to sound too deep it's a purpose. To share this way of life with womankind. I've also had participants who have been so inspired that they've chosen to train in fitness and pass on the message. Now that's inspiring. More on that later.

I'm not just a fitness megalomaniac

So that's me! And I think that's really all you need for now. I just wanted to put in a bit of context so you know I'm not just a fitness megalomaniac. I have a soul and I've had life shocks too. But I believe you can use them to make something amazing happen in your life. I could have felt sorry for myself and I understand that for some, their go to safe place might be food or self harm (have you considered eating could be a form of self-harm)? But you can turn things around with a little support. So perhaps you've had a major life shock which has triggered depression, emotional eating or self-sabotage and you can't get out of it. I'll go into more on this later but just know for now that your trigger foods are addictive and will help to bury you in your hole. You need to break the chain. How about it?

Untruths and myths about diets

I'm going to start by breaking down the biggest untruths and myths about diets whilst sharing with you some important truths that aren't getting out there.

You see I've been in the fitness industry a while now. I was doing it back in the 80s and 90s when aerobics was in, along with fluoro unitards, Pineapple one pieces, flesh coloured tights and slouch socks. Yes, I've lived the 80s fitness dream!

The low fat zone

Back in the 80s and 90s, we were in the low fat zone. I was teaching around 30 classes a week, seven days a week and presenting at the weekends. I ate low fat. My average day consisted of porridge for breakfast, a jacket potato for lunch plus and apple and a yoghurt as snacks. Then I would eat late, after classes. That was the dieting era when cottage cheese ruled the supermarket shelves and we all got indigestion!

But for all my sweating and low fat eating I was fat. Not fat as in overweight or obese but - and you see this a lot with fitness instructors - almost like a chiseled marshmallow. Back in the early 90s it was more like a sweaty marshmallow in slouch socks.

Year on year I was putting on more weight. I'd do more classes and I'd do more training but I'd still get fatter. I was a typical aerobics instructor. I'd got definition and decent legs but always carried it round my middle.

And here's why this is all relevant. I wanted to know why after years of a low fat diet with lots of exercise I wasn't a stick. Wouldn't you? I mean, after years of trying the diet that should get you lean and instead getting fatter (and I really wasn't cheating on the low fat thing) you'd want to know why wouldn't you?

Failure to reach your target weight or size is not altogether your fault
I can't stress enough how much the failure to reach your target weight or size is not altogether your fault. It's just that you've never been given the right information or the right tools. This is why I'm writing this book.

Cortisol

I thought that by teaching 30 classes a week, doing my own training and eating what I thought was a 'healthy' diet (low fat, high carbohydrate meals and snacks) I should lose weight. But year on year I was consistently putting weight on. To be precise, the weight was going on around my middle and I couldn't understand it.

I thought I was doing EVERYTHING right until I started to research cortisol. From what I then learned about cortisol I realised I was doing everything to confuse this otherwise clever hormone!

Cortisol is a naturally occurring hormone.[2] Think of it as your stress hormone. It's released into the bloodstream in response to stress or a low level of blood glucocorticoid (a type of

---

[2] Cortisol is a steroid hormone, a glucocorticoid produced by the zona fasisculata of the adrenal cortex.

hormone) and plays a vital role in increasing blood sugar, suppressing the immune system and helping to metabolise fats, protein and carbohydrates. It's part of the fight or flight response, preparing your body for rapid action. In short, cortisol helps to give us high energy for a few hours then crashes.

Cortisol isn't all bad. It's naturally high in the morning, to give us a little get up and go and should wain by the evening to ensure a good night's sleep. But with our hectic, 24-hour lifestyles, grazing habits and eating on-the-go, poor quality sleep and high sugar and fructose intake, our cortisol levels can get out of whack.

Cortisol regulation is important for dieters

Cortisol regulation is important for dieters because too much, too often is a major factor in laying down fat around our middles (Moyer, 1994).[3] Whenever your cortisol levels are high and you don't need extra energy, you're encouraging fatty deposits around your tummy.

It's not just about the way we look, those fat deposits go down around our internal organs and it's this visceral fat which is so bad for our health. Fatty deposits around our internal organs increase our risk of type 2 diabetes (Gastaldellii 2008).[4]

These fatty deposits also put us at greater risk of high blood pressure. A 2014 study found the visceral fat rather than Body Mass Index (BMI) or overall subcutaneous fat (the fat around our organs) was associated with an increased risk of developing high blood pressure (Chandra 2014).[5] Subcutaneous fat has also been linked to a higher risk of heart disease, stroke and colorectal cancer and the only thing that can shift this type of fat is lifestyle change.

Cortisol makes slim women fat

A 2000 study from Yale University found that even slim women may be carrying excess visceral abdominal fat due to the effects of stress (Epel, 2000).[6] The study specifically linked abdominal fat to cortisol rather than just stress, suggesting that it was the levels of cortisol in women's bodies and their sensitivity to it which led to fatty deposits.

As you've probably guessed, there is more to raised cortisol than stress alone. Every time you eat or snack during the day your cortisol is raised. Over exercising, such as performing low intensity, steady state exercise like long distance running can increase it.[7] Poor quality sleep and high carbohydrate diets can all leave your bloodstream with constantly high levels of cortisol.

---

[3] Moyer, AE (May 1994) *'Stress-induced cortisol response and fat distribution in women.'* Obesity Research & Clinical Practice Journal 2(3), p255-62

[4] Gastaldellii, A. (May 2008) *'Abdominal fat: does it predict the development of type 2 diabetes?'* American Journal of Clinical Nutrition, vol. 87,no. 5, p1118-1119.

[5] Chandra, A, et al (2014) *'The relationship of body mass and fat distribution with incident hypertension',* Journal of the American College of Cardiology 64; pp997-1002.

[6] Epel. E (2000) *'Stress and Body Shape: Stress-Induced Cortisol Secretion Is Consistently Greater Among Women With Central Fat'*, Psychosomatic Medicine 62; pp623-632

[7] Some studies have suggested that over time, the increased cortisol brought on by endurance exercise will level out and your body may be able to cope with it better.

Fat is your body's way of telling you something isn't right

There is lots you can do to regulate cortisol and cut down your disease risk. The side effect of this is often fat loss.

It's fantastic that today's society is so much more accepting of different body shapes and sizes but we can't forget that excess fat is your body's way of telling you something isn't right.

Cutting Calories

The majority of diets involve calorie restriction in some way. It's just the way it's always been done.

But calorie restriction just makes you hungry and grumpy.

Hunger decreases your mental and physical performance and makes you cranky.

Cutting calories makes you tired and unproductive.

It's little wonder that most people give up on diets. Why wouldn't you crave those foods that make you feel good, even if it's just for a little while?

Being hungry is not a sign of mental toughness. It's torture!

In my opinion, the diet and nutrition news that gets into mainstream media is, at best, about five years out of date. If you want to know the facts about how you could get the body you want and deserve then stick with me. If you want to know how and why women across the UK are dropping not just pounds but stones, please hear me out.

The diet and willpower myth

Many diets would have you believe that if you can't stick to them, you and your lack of willpower are in some way to blame. Or that you aren't trying hard enough.

Foods like wheat, gluten and sugar are addictive (I'll explain more on this later). They give you a temporary high but leave you craving more a few hours later. Imagine cutting calories but still needing those addictive foods.

Kick Start Fat Loss can break the willpower battle. By consuming foods that leave you satisfied and break food addictions you will be satiated for longer, which could help prevent those temporary feel good food cravings.

Eating good fats like butter and coconut oil, getting your carbohydrates from great, non-addictive sources and eating a moderate to high protein diet on a regular basis will leave your body satisfied and give you energy rather than a bad case of the hunger crankiness.

Fat Phobia

Are you fat phobic?

Do you believe that eating fat will make you fat?

Fat has a bad reputation. But what about the good things?

- Fats add flavour to food and keep you fuller for longer.
- Some fats help you to burn fat.
- Fats are essential for brain function.
- Fats keep our brains and bodies healthy (some fats are used to help manage Alzheimer's disease and epilepsy).
- Fats are essential for hormone regulation and function.
- Vitamins A, E, D and K are fat soluble vitamins. So we need fat for these nutrients.
- We can't produce Omega 3 so need to consume it through our fat intake.
- You don't gain fat by eating fat.

Do you know that the low fat movement was largely driven by the researcher Ancel Keys and the work he did in the middle of last century? Low fat diets are literally a hangover from the 1970s Seven Countries Study (Keys, 1970).[8]

Fat and Coronary Heart Disease (CHD)
We went low fat because Keys (amongst others) discovered a link between CHD and high fat diets. Dubbed, the 'lipid theory' of heart disease, his study found that in countries where dietary fat intake was high and a component of every meal there was a strong link to higher mortality rates through CHD and high cholesterol levels. The opposite was also true.

Do you remember the Mediterranean Diet? That was Keys following the Seven Countries Study.

How about Statins? Keys triggered them too.

This low fat ideology was promoted by doctors and governments (so we all believed it).

Meanwhile, we ignored sugar and the food industry got busy finding tasty alternatives to fat, which often meant adding sugar or sweeteners to give the food back the taste that taking the fat out took away!

Keys discredited
Earlier this year The British Medical Journal (BMJ) published a new meta-analysis looking at the randomised controlled trials (RCTs) that were available to US and UK committees in the 1970s when they introduced low fat, government guidelines (Harcombe, 2015).[9] The

----

[8] Keys. A (1970) *Coronary Heart Disease in Seven Countries.*

[9] Harcombe. Z (2015) '*Evidence from randomised controlled trials did not support the introduction of dietary fat guidelines in 1977 and 1983: a systematic review and meta-analysis.*" Open Heart 2: doi:10.1136/openhrt-2014-000196

study was undertaken because no-one had studied the evidence base for recommending low fat diets.

The study concluded that low fat guidelines were introduced without supporting evidence from RCTs.

Last year the US *Time Magazine* did a complete about face on the 'lipid theory' of heart disease. They admitted they were wrong. *Time Magazine* had led the media charge against saturated fats in the 1970s and 1980s.

Saturated fat is not the enemy.

Stable fat
Saturated facts are in fact stable fats compared with polyunsaturated fats (those fats like margarine and vegetable oil which we were 'told' were healthy). A stable fat is a fat which is less likely to go rancid or oxidise. This makes it easier to cook with and much better for our health. An oil which is unstable or goes rancid easily is more likely to be unhealthy, causing damage to the body at a cellular level.

Stable fats are the least inflammatory macro nutrient, so brilliant for a healthy gut and body.[10] Fats like butter from grass fed cows and coconut oil are great sources, or raw olive oil and avocados. Precisely those foods that many low fat diets recommend you cut out or cut down on.

Polyunsaturated fats
The polyunsaturated fats to avoid are oils like Canola, corn, peanut, soya or vegetable oils. From a very practical point of view it is much harder to extract oil from a vegetable than it is from cow's milk. So not only is the oil itself less stable but also more highly processed than saturated fats.

Butter
On the *Kick Start Fat Loss* detox we eliminate all dairy from the diet except for butter. Milk proteins are largely absent in butter and the little milk protein that remains in cultured butter has been modified during the butter fermentation process making it tolerant for most people.

Grass fed cow's milk in butter
The secret ingredient in butter that is made from grass fed cows is Butyrate. This is the same compound your gut bacteria produces.

Butyrate is a short chain saturated fatty acid and in humans has been proven to reduce inflammation and keep toxins from penetrating the gut lining.

Butter is a health food!
However it is important to consume the right butter.

---

[10] Macro nutrients are protein, carbohydrates and fat.

In order to provide you with Vitamin A, K2, D & E the butter must be from grass fed cows and if possible organic, from a local farm where the cows have eaten a healthy diet free from GM ingredients, free from antibiotics and growth hormones.

Things to look out for when choosing your butter:

Is the butter from grass fed cows? Butter from grass fed cows (even 90%) still contains higher quantities of omega-3. Also cows are not given antibiotics or growth hormones.

Milk from cows that are grass-fed is rich in natural beta-carotene.

Is the butter made from milk where cows are bovine somatotropin (rBGH producing supplemental hormone) free?

Confirm that the butter itself is free of GM ingredients.

If you cannot tolerate butter or are allergic to casein or lactose then try Ghee (clarified butter).

Kick Start LOVE Calon Wen Organic Unsalted Butter.

Coconut Oil

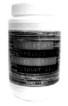

If you've yet to discover coconut oil this is one ingredient you need to have in your cupboard.

Coconut oil contains a type of saturated fat that the body processes differently to other types of saturated fact and is very good for you.

Coconut oil is the richest source of saturated fat known to man (90% saturated).

Why Coconut Oil Is So Good For You?
The form of fat that's found in coconut oil is referred to as medium chain triglycerides (MCTs). MCTs can increase energy expenditure compared with other fats, so they literally help you to burn calories.

One study found that 15-30 grams of MCTs per day increased 24 hour energy expenditure by 5%, totalling about 120 calories per day (Dulloo, 1996).[11]

Medium Chain Triglycerides (MCTs)
MCTs are used immediately as energy for the body, just as carbohydrates would be. Therefore, for those on low carbohydrate diets, MCTs can be a very powerful weapon and act in your favour. MCTs are also important for brain health and have been used to help brain disorders like Alzheimer's.

---

[11] Dulloo. AG (1996) "*Twenty-four-hour energy expenditure and urinary catecholamines of humans consuming low-to-moderate amounts of medium-chain triglycerides: a dose-response study in a human respiratory chamber.*" European Journal of Clinical Nutrition 50(3); pp152-8.

Coconut oil can also improve your cholesterol levels by increasing the amount of good cholesterol (HDL) in your blood.

Regular use of coconut oil can help you to recover faster after workouts and reduce your susceptibility to common colds. The lauric acid in coconut oil is converted to monolaurin which has anti-bacterial and anti-viral properties so it can give your immune system a boost.

Moisture
Not only will coconut oil add moisture to your food but it's great for skin, nails and hair too or just used as a moisturiser.

How to cook with coconut oil
Coconut oil can be used as an easy replacement for other oils in cooking and is particularly good at high temperatures. It's great in stir-fries, sauces, roasting or baking recipes. You can also add it smoothies to make them naturally sweet and creamy.

Facts about dieting and fat loss

So we've tackled cortisol, low fat and types of fat. For me, these are the biggest players when it comes to dieting falsehoods. But what of those little myths you hear at work, on the radio or, 'from your mam?' Those things you just believe and which form the foundation of your weight loss mission.

Well we've got those covered too.

'I just need to do more exercise.'
You don't. You just need to workout smarter. More exercise does not always correlate to fat reduction. Some studies have shown that long duration, low intensity exercise like long distance running could increase your cortisol levels (Balsalobre-Fernández, 2014).[12] Also consider what you're more able to achieve, a 10 minute workout every day or a 60 minute one?

Kick Start Fat Loss workouts are based on High Intensity Interval Training (HIIT), where you workout as hard as you can in short bursts during one ten minute workout. According to a 2011 study presented at the American College of Sports Medicine Annual Meeting, just two weeks of high-intensity intervals improves your aerobic capacity as much as six to eight weeks of endurance training (Ziemann et al, 2011).[13] And interval training like this will leave you burning fat for up to 24 hours after your workout.[14]

'I know I need to eat little and often to keep my metabolism high.'
This is a myth. Unless you are training for a marathon or an endurance event you do not need to eat throughout the day. There is no evidence to support this dieting trend. Grazing is a massive problem for women. Eating little and often becomes eating a lot often. It can often contribute to over eating.

'I just need to switch all my normal foods to low fat or diet options.'
Please do not do this! Later in the book I'll explain why diet foods are trapping you in a dieting cycle and how to break it - for good - but for now, it is a fact that you do not need to eat low fat to get lean. Like any processed foods, processed diet foods can be low in nutrients and packed with hidden sugars (because of the amount of time they have to spend on the shelves) - again, there's more on this later. Use fresh, unprocessed ingredients and cook from scratch wherever possible.

'I just need to swap my lunch for a bowl of cereal.'
In *Kick Start Fat Loss* we ban all breakfast cereals, even if they are marketed as healthy. Yes many are low in calories and yes many are low in fat but breakfast cereals are processed grains. If you are trying to lose weight and get more energy by regulating your hormones, especially insulin and cortisol, a big bowl of what the body regards as processed carbohydrates (or sugar) isn't the best place to start. If you try to eat only breakfast cereals you'll just be hungry.

---

[12]Balsalobre-Fernández, C. (2014) *'Hormonal and neuromuscular responses to high-level middle- and long-distance competition.'* International Journal of Sport Phyiology and Performance, Sep: 9(5):839-44

[13] Ziemann, E. (2011) *'Aerobic and Anaerobic Changes with High Intensity Interval Training in Active College Aged Men.'* The Journal of Strength and Conditioning Research, Apr: 1104-1112

[14] Trainers refer to this phenomenon as excess post exercise oxygen consumption (or EPOC).

'I know I should be keeping an eye on my calories.'
Don't count calories. All calories are not equal. I'll explain all about this in the Diet Detox chapter. Go for high quality fresh vegetables, meat and fish (organic where possible).

'I need to ditch the holistic stuff in the gym and just go for the burn.'
10 minutes of yoga, Pilates or meditation will not burn fat BUT it will help you to de-stress and produce less cortisol. This can make you leaner, less stressed and let's face it, happier - which is after all the end goal.

'I've heard fasting will lower my metabolism.'
There's no evidence to suggest your metabolic rate will drop if you fast. Fasting can be beneficial for fat loss.

Some studies also point to fasted training (not eating before you exercise or exercising first thing in the morning) as a brilliant way of encouraging your body to use fat as fuel (Gonzalez, 2013).[15] It's a training protocol that's been used for years by body builders needing to get lean for an event or actors getting in shape for a film.

And whilst we're on the subject of fasting, you don't have to eat breakfast the minute you get up. If you prefer to eat your first meal of the day at 11 o'clock this is fine, it will not slow down your metabolism.

'I simply can't lose weight.'
You can. This is where mental fitness comes into it - a big part of *Kick Start Fat Loss*. If you can change your mind chatter and be positive, it will help you to get leaner. The first step to a a more fabulous you is to stop mentally beating yourself up. I recently interviewed one of *Kick Start Fat Loss*'s biggest losers, Lesley Gooch, who has just passed the nine stone fat loss mark (you've already heard from Lesley). When I asked her what the biggest change was she said it was realising that the dieting industry was lying to her. Low fat, low calorie and slimming clubs she'd tried before were trapping her in her fat body. Later in the book we'll discuss becoming your own food and diet detective.

'I don't have time to cook.'
If there's one thing I urge you to do it's to find a love of food preparation. It is the only way to ensure your diet is sugar, preservative and chemical free. It could be salads. It could be as simple as a chicken breast with a pile of vegetables or salad but please ditch the microwave and ready meals and cook from scratch. I've included lots of recipe suggestions in the book and there are many more ideas online.

---

[15] Gonzalez. J, Veasey. R, Rumbold. S, Stevenson. E (2013). *'Breakfast and exercise contingently affect postprandial metabolism and energy balance in physically active males.' British Journal of Nutrition,* 110, pp 721-732.

Kim Lee

Kim started *Kick Start Fat Loss* in West Wickham, in April 2013. Kim was afraid of what people would think of her and also how much time she'd have to spend cooking from scratch (something she rarely, if ever did). Kim is another of *Kick Start Fat Loss'*s massive success stories. She has not only transformed her lifestyle but Kim has finally, following her weight loss, been given the go ahead to have the breast reduction surgery she has always wanted. Kim is 40 and lives in Croydon. Here is Kim's *Kick Start Fat Loss* story:

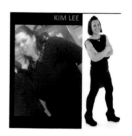

I've always been self-conscious of my size, especially of my big boobs and would wear big, baggy tops to cover up. I notice at school that it's usually the bigger girls who drop out of sports or feel embarrassed and I know that feeling. I can see their point of view. I used to think that people would laugh at me if I exercised. It's so embarrassing. You think that people are staring. Your confidence is zero.

I'd tried all the usual diets before. Weight watchers, Slimming World, the Cambridge Diet, the Cabbage Soup Diet but I'd only ever lost a couple of pounds here and there. So after weeks of nagging from my cousin I eventually went along to my first Kick Start Fat Loss session. To be honest, I just went to shut her up.

When I went to my first session I felt sick. I had bad butterflies in my stomach. I made every excuse not to go. I thought the instructor would judge me and that everyone would stare at me. "Look at her, the new one. What's she doing?" But it was the complete opposite. I felt like part of the team. I felt included.

When I started Kick Start Fat Loss I was 15 stone 12 pounds. I was a size 18-20 bottom and 24-26 top.

In the first week I lost seven pounds. "Actually this is working," I thought. After four weeks I'd lost 18 pounds.

I knew I had to change the way I ate in order to make a difference. I think a big change was turning 40 and realising I wasn't young anymore. I was more focused than I'd ever been before and the constant encouragement from the Kick Start Fat Loss team kept me going. Plus my children are older so no longer needed constant attention. I have five children, my youngest is eight and my eldest is 19. It was my time and I'd never really had that before.

When I started Kick Start Fat Loss I told them, "you'll still get quality time. Life will be better," and it is. I now go to keep fit three times a week and I go jogging a lot. They understand why.

If I'm honest, looking back to before Kick Start Fat Loss I couldn't really walk. I thought I was exercising but I just waddled everywhere. So when I started Kick Start Fat Loss I took it all at my own pace. I couldn't do certain exercises. Now I can do them all, I can even do a full press up and I'm training to be a fitness instructor.

I've lost nearly six stones in total. I'm now a size 10-12 in trousers and a 12-14 top. Before Kick Start Fat Loss I hated shopping. Now I love it!

My children are all really proud of what I've achieved and tell me on a daily basis. It gives me goosebumps. Although the older ones don't like that I can now borrow their clothes!

I've seen a massive change in the health of our whole family because of the new way we eat. My eldest daughter was overweight last year and my other children were probably borderline. My daughter had pretty bad eczema which has nearly cleared up and another daughter has asthma which has really improved. We rarely get ill anymore. Our skin is better, our hair is better, it's shiny and in good condition. Our faces are glowing, we just look healthy.

And from being a lazy cook, I now spend quality time with my children cooking. We cook everything from scratch. The children also take it in turns to cook, they like to see what's going in their food and have really taken an interest in meals.

Every time I look back now at what I used to do and what I used to eat I just cringe. We would have takeaways two or three times a week and the cupboards were full of crisps and chocolate.

I just don't have it around now, I don't have it in the cupboards.

The biggest change for me has been no coffee. I used to drink a lot but I haven't had any coffee since I started.

There's no pasta or potatoes either and no bags of crisps. But now I don't want to eat any of those things. Instead I now enjoy things like spinach and courgettes, which I never used to eat. And we've changed from normal milk to almond milk and coconut milk. It's a complete turnaround.

When I started I didn't really have a main goal, I just knew I needed to lose weight. But honestly, I've always wanted a breast reduction but have never had the confidence to go to the doctor about it. So last summer, I plucked up the courage to go and see my doctor. My Kick Start Fat Loss coach Chris had been really supportive and encouraged me to go.

The doctor was really understanding and referred me to the hospital. At the hospital appointment I was told I needed to lose another two stone in order to have the surgery. I'm pretty sure they told me this never expecting me to lose the weight. That made me even more determined. I needed to do it for me!

Even though I'd lost the weight, I still got the back aches and my shoulders hurt but now I knew it was my boobs and not all the extra weight I'd been carrying.

I've now got the go ahead for the surgery!"

I fit my fitness trainer studies around my job as a teaching assistant. I plan on taking over some of Chris's classes and launching my own in Croydon. I'd also like to bring exercise into my school and pass on what I've learned to the pupils and staff there through PE lessons and after school clubs.

Kick Start Fat Loss is a lifestyle change. Come and give it a try, it works. You can make all the excuses you want but your excuses will eventually run out.

Victoria Brodie-Smith

Slimming clubs. The cabbage soup detox. The egg and grapefruit diet. Slimming pills. These are just some of the many diets tried and tested by London based health care assistant Victoria Brodie-Smith. At the start of her weight loss journey Victoria weighed 12 stone 8lbs. She wanted to put a stop to her 'serial dieting' and find a solution to her sugar addiction. Victoria joined *Kick Start Fat Loss* Mill Hill and Barnet, run by franchisee Esther Shortt in ....

This is Victoria's three and a half stone *Kick Start Fat Loss* story:

Before Kick Start Fat Loss my diet was heavy on sugar and carbohydrates. Now I eat nutrient rich foods like scrambled egg with smoked salmon, tomato and spinach for breakfast; a big salad for lunch; and meat or fish with vegetables for dinner.

I love the simplicity of it and the way it keeps me full. I was known in the past for being hungry all the time. I now know that was the sugar in all the diet foods I ate.

By combining healthy home cooked meals and regular exercise - including kettlebells and Zumba - I've seen a steady weight loss of three and half stone over nine months. I feel great. I'm more confident, I have more energy, I don't get out of breath any more and I know I look nice in clothes now.

I couldn't have been so successful without both the one to one support from my coach Esther and the online support from the Kick Start Fat Loss Facebook page. All the members post pictures of their meals and give advice where needed. It's a great way to source ideas and the support has been invaluable.

If you want to break free from the diet trap you have to go back to basics. Forget processed food or anything that has been through a process. Stick with food that is in its most natural state. If you can't grow it or rear it, then don't eat it."

About Kick Start Fat Loss

Kick Start Fat Loss was created in response to new and evolving nutritional research.

In the past 20 years we have got fatter and fatter and are now in the midst of a world wide health epidemic.

In the UK alone, obesity among adults has increased sharply since the 1990s. From 13.2% of men and 16.4% of women in 1993, to 24.2% of men and 25.1% of women in 2012 (Health Survey for England, 2013).[16] By 2050 obesity is predicted to affect 60% of adult men, 50% of adult women and 25% of children (Reducing Obesity: Future Choices, 2007).[17]

Yet over the same period nutritional and dieting advice has remained constant.

We've got fatter
So perhaps this is why, whilst we haven't been listening, we've got fatter. This is why, whilst I was exercising my little bottom off and eating low fat I was still fat and getting fatter.

Women are still accepting the same diet and nutrition advice
As a nation we have got fatter by listening to the same advice - and yet people I meet are still resistant to change.

They are still resistant to doing things differently.

Why is that the case when it hasn't worked?

I find it really strange that intelligent women, women who are smashing through boundaries in their careers or starting up their own businesses whilst managing a family too - really amazing women - are still accepting the same diet and nutrition advice. Take a look around any mummy group on Facebook and the same few slimming clubs are discussed.

If super smart, switched on women aren't getting it, then there must be some serious marketing, advertising tricks that are really working. Something subliminal, dare I say perhaps even multi-million pound brainwashing.

Let's pause a little on that.

We'll go into food and diet marketing tricks when we discuss your mind set and how you can be your own food detective. We're going to start with the external stuff which you can consciously control.

---

[16] *Health Survey for England* (2012) available from http://www.hscic.gov.uk/catalogue/PUB13218

[17] *Reducing Obesity: Future Choices* (Oct 2007), part of Foresight Projects, Government Office for Science, available from https://www.gov.uk/government/publications/reducing-obesity-future-choices

What diets are out there?

Before we get started on the *Kick Start Fat Loss* plan, I want to explore the most common diets that are around at the moment. They aren't all bad. There are good points and bad points to everything but I know that if I'm asking you to disregard much of what you've held to be true about dieting for so long, you'll probably take some convincing.

How do I know this? Because everyone that walks into my *Kick Start Fat Loss* classes for the first time feels the same way.

Calorie controlled diets
Any diet will work for a short time and calorie controlled diets are no exception.

Calorie controlled diets are often well structured and easy to follow. You don't have to change your food groups or the way that you eat, you just eat less or buy low calorie options - so they fit easily into your life. You also don't have to exercise to start getting results.

These diets can also appear very convenient for busy people, like working mums or new mums who are struggling enough to keep children and themselves alive let alone plan a radical eating regime.

Calorie controlled diets are however difficult to sustain for a long period of time. Also, by limiting your calorie intake you are often limiting your nutritional intake, especially good fats from sources like avocado, nuts and oily fish. And if we return to our busy mum or executive population, they are precisely the people who need good fats to help brain function and mood.

Without exercise and with a limited calorie intake, calorie controlled diets can put you at risk of losing muscle mass, a big limitation for long term weight maintenance and long term health.

Calorie controlled diets often appeal to an older age demographic, who are already at risk of losing muscle mass. Dieting like this on a regular basis can leave dieters weak and out of shape.

Calorie controlled diets can also really sap the pleasure out of eating. You are still addicted to processed, sugary foods and not exposed to a great variety. You get used to knowing what you can eat and what is a 'bad' food.

There are numerous studies which have proven that in the long run, dieters who do calorie controlled diets put the weight back on and more after they finish the diet. Not only is it not a long term solution but it could be argued they are bad for your health by restricting your nutritional intake and affecting percentage of lean tissue to fatty tissue in your body.

Fasting or intermittent fasting
Let's get this out there first: Fasting will not lower your metabolism. In fact, fasting can be a really effective tool in your fat loss box. For starters, it gives your digestive system a complete rest.[18]

---

[18] I'm defining fasting as controlled periods with absolutely no food rather than calorie controlled starvation.

Fasting may also encourage your body to use fat stores for fuel (Gonzalez, 2013).

It can also help you to burn fat easier by making you more sensitive to insulin. When you don't eat, you don't produce insulin to break down food, therefore you become more sensitive to insulin which makes fat loss easier. Being sensitive to insulin is much better for our health, long term.

On a psychological level, fasting helps you to mentally unchain your self from food, so is especially useful if you are an emotional eater or eat when you're bored. Go on a fast and you'll soon notice when you're actually hungry compared with what your mind is telling you about why you think you should eat.

And, on a practical level, fasting frees up more time!

A quick note on this though, fasting is not suitable for anyone who has ever suffered with or is still suffering from an eating disorder - especially those involving starvation.

On the down side, uncontrolled fasting can lead to binge eating. You need to really prepare yourself, your cupboards and your fridge.

The most effective way to break from a fast is with a greens drink or juice and to eat clean.

Blood type diet

The blood type diet is - as the name suggests - based on your blood type. The diet creators believe that by eating according to your blood group, you'll lose weight, feel healthier and reduce your risk of disease. Celebrities like Cheryl Cole, Liz Hurley and Courtney Cox-Arquette are reported to have got great results from the Blood Type Diet.

The blood type diet premise is that your optimal nutritional intake can be found from knowing your blood group. And different blood groups need different foods.

I wouldn't however, advocate this unless you've had a full food sensitivity blood test. A full blood test (not just one that tells you your blood group) is the only way to get a true picture of what foods you are sensitive too.

The best thing about the blood type diet is that it does encourage everyone to exercise, regardless of blood group. But it is very complicated and time consuming and could put you at risk of reducing your nutrient variety by limiting your diet to your blood group.

Food combining

There are several diets that might fall into this category. The Hay Diet is probably the most famous one. What they have in common is the fact that they are designed to stimulate your metabolism and to make sure that you burn fat quickly and effectively.

The most important 'rule' with most food combining diets is that protein, like meats and beans, should not be combined with starches, like bread, rice, and pasta. Fruits should be eaten on their own, and proteins and starches should be paired up with other vegetables.

There are some great things about food combining diets. Firstly, you don't have to cut anything major from your diet. For instance, you don't have to give up starches (like you do with the Atkins diet). You'll also find that when you really give your all to a food combining diet you'll become much better at planning your meals. This can and usually will help you make healthier choices. Food planning is also great for your budget!

Whilst some people report great results from food combining, there isn't a great deal of research behind it. In my opinion it's possible that results come more from food planning and preparation than the food combining element.

Meal replacement diets

We all know about those meal replacement diets. And I'm sure we all know someone who has been on one or perhaps is on one.

The concept of a 'nutrition bullet' meal replacement diet can be appealing to time starved people.

It's understandable. There's no need to worry about shopping or cooking, you just put your trust into a meal replacement shake or similar and magically lose weight. It's convenient and seems too good to be true, especially when there are miraculous weight loss case studies to support some products.

The major downside of meal replacement diet products is the post diet binge. Like all calorie controlled diets, the urge to eat after what seems like starvation to your body is strong and the drastic weight loss is not sustainable long term.

The other issue I have with meal replacement diets is the highly processed, high sugar or sugar substitute content of some shakes. Sugar and many sugar substitutes are addictive (more on this in the next chapter).

The effects of our external environment on our health

Scientists and in turn fitness and health professionals are beginning to understand more about our bodies, specifically the way we metabolize food and the ways in which we are affected by our external environment.

As a result, we are now better equipped to tackle fat loss and major health conditions from a nutritional and lifestyle perspective.

Our weight and health is not only dictated by what we put into our mouths but by what we put onto our skin, surround ourselves with and ultimately consume.

Pollutants, stress, sleep, food and beauty product preservatives, cheap food and chemicals all affect our health and the way our bodies store fat. Then there's the amount of time we spend on our mobile phones or the internet, the way we cook or store our food, not to mention hidden sugars and chemicals. Even our bank balances and the great British climate have a part to play in how we store fat and of course, how we feel about ourselves.

It is virtually impossible to fix everything in our environments but if you consider how much is working against you, it gives you a clue as to why you have yet to achieve your ideal weight. Even if it was all about counting calories (which I can assure you it isn't), with everything else working against you, you'd still be fighting a losing battle. So give yourself a break!

We cannot change hereditary factors which affect our health but we can control many environmental factors, such as the chemicals we put on our bodies. We can control the amount of exercise and the quality of exercise we perform and we can control what we put into our mouths, how we prepare our food and the quality of food we buy.

If there is so much stacked against you and your endeavors AND your dieting advice is, at best, flawed, how have you stood a chance? Until now that is ...

You aren't just what you eat, you are what you absorb too.

Let's break this down a little more. What's changed in the last 20 years?

There are more cars on the road
This contributes to airborne pollution from petrol and diesel fumes which we inhale and which also sit on our skin, lungs and on the farm crops we eat. Aside from carbon monoxide there are multiple pollutants in exhaust fumes which can harm us.

Poor farming weather
From climate change and chemicals to cost cuts in farming, the food we buy and eat has changed and is still changing. Mass production of crops and meat and a demand for reduced costs has contributed to a change in the quality of some of the foods we eat.

Increase in pharmaceutical drugs
We are taking more tablets than ever before.

More cleaning agents
Take a look around your home (usually under your sink). How many products do you use? There is some evidence to suggest that trace chemicals in some cleaning products may affect our endrocrine (hormonal) systems.

Increased environmental contaminants
Pesticides and herbicides do a great job of keeping insects off crops. They are also impossible to wash off. Eating only a small amount can affect your body's delicate balance. Even an organic farm cannot have pure organic produce. If the environment's toxicity level is high, the air will carry gasses. We can only reduce contaminants, we can't eliminate them completely.

We want to look fit, not be fit.
We have a lazy nation that is not getting fitter. Statistics show the problem isn't unique to adults, it starts with our children. The latest figures from the National Child Measurement Programme (NCMP) for 2013/14 show that a third of 10-11 year olds and over a fifth of 4-5 year olds were overweight or obese. Unfortunately, many view health and fitness as a social trend rather then part of a lifestyle. Statistically gym attendance booms in January, April and September. Why? New year's resolutions, summer holiday preparation, post holiday reparations and Christmas booty training. The truth is that we want to look fit, not be fit!

Increased use of technology
The internet is now a crucial part of our lifestyle. We have information and communication at our fingertips as well as online shopping and remote working opportunities. This convenience gives us even fewer reasons to leave the house and move our bodies.

Artificial preservatives
Preservatives in food increases its shelf life, thereby making it cheaper (less waste). All food is subjected to air and starts a process called oxidisation. This in time creates free radicals. Free radicals have been linked with diseases like cancer because they are extremely reactive and can cause cell damage in the body. Fresh food like vegetables and grass fed meat do not contain these.

Importation of cheaper foods
It has become cheaper to import food internationally because cost and consumer demand. Transportation times are long reducing freshness of foods and increasing the need for pesticides and preservatives.

Increased alcohol consumption
We are drinking more than before. This increases our intake of toxins and sugars.

Increased sugar consumption
The amount of sugar we consume has increased. Sugars are hidden in drinks, sweeteners, sauces, energy and sports drinks and in low fat foods as well as many processed foods.

Increased fast and convenience foods
As we get busier, we need quicker options for food. So we often turn to fast food or ready meals. This means we are consuming more highly processed foods.

Increase in sedentary/office jobs
We sit down for long periods. The average person stands for no more than two hours per day in total.

Detoxify your body

Kick Start Fat Loss is a very simple programme based on cooking from scratch and using natural and organic ingredients wherever possible. It starts with a 28 day 'clean eating' detox. This doesn't mean you have to buy or drink any disgusting potions, or a week of super teenage acne but it does mean eliminating all processed foods, coffee, tea, alcohol, sugar, and ready meals from your diet.

Detoxifying the body, liver, and cells will help the body burn fat more efficiently, becoming leaner and stronger. This might sound tough but it gets results, establishes great habits and will motivate you to keep going.

Dairy, gluten, sugar, alcohol and caffeine
Dairy, gluten, sugar, alcohol and caffeine are some of the most common culprits for irritation or creating inflammation in the body. This is the main reason we eliminate these from the diet. If the thought of this fills you with fear then you could consider eliminating one thing at a time over a period of weeks and months. Your results will be slower but if it works better for you, there's no reason why you can't do it this way.

In 14 days you can completely detoxify the body
If you commit to it, in 14 days you can completely detoxify the body. We start with a 28 day detox because this is the optimum amount of time to get your body healthy and ready for the fat loss programme (although most of my participants have their biggest fat and inch losses during the initial 28 day detox).

The aims of the first 28 day of *Kick Start Fat Loss* are:

1. To break the body's addiction to sugar.
2. To detoxify the body and cells so fat is burned more effectively.
3. To regulate blood sugar throughout the day to stop craving high fat, high carbohydrate foods.
4. To begin to enjoy cooking from scratch with whole, natural and seasonal foods and ingredients.
5. To stop grazing.
6. To understand and appreciate the importance of vegetables in the war against body fat.
7. To give you unlimited energy.
8. To lose body fat and inches.

Natasha Knight

Natasha has been a *Kick Start Fat Loss* franchise holder since 2013. She is based in North London (N8 and N22). Natasha was a fitness instructor before starting with *Kick Start Fat Loss* but she transformed her body from fit to super fit and lean with the *Kick Start Fat Loss* detox and programme. Natasha has also boosted her business and business profile through *Kick Start Fat Loss*. She says her confidence has gone through the roof. Natasha is 42 and lives in London. Here's Natasha's *Kick Start Fat Loss* story:

I had been looking at Kick Start Fat Loss for a while but thought, "it's not for me - I'm not into all the clean eating. I'm a hard core fitness trainer." I knew a bit about nutrition. Well thought I did!

I've been self employed for years. Working for studios and dabbling with my own classes. I ran bootcamps and Zumba classes successfully but I felt like I could never do it on my own. All I knew was to work really hard, long hours. I'm a grafter by nature but before I started Kick Start Fat Loss I felt like I was just going round in circles. I was literally on my knees. I had no motivation for work. I knew I needed direction and support.

Eventually I emailed Rachel. In fact I emailed her about five times! Until after lots of excuses and lots of anxiety I decided to just jump. Take a risk Tasha! I trusted Rachel and I needed help and direction.

So I joined up and nearly had a nervous breakdown. Wow! As I prepared to change my mindset lots of feelings came bubbling up. This was a huge deal for me and to be honest I didn't really know what I was getting into - I tend to just do things that feel right.

Kick Start Fat Loss pushed me out of my comfort zone. In becoming a franchisee I had to look at my career and business model honestly. It was like peeling layers of an onion away and still is.

As for the the detox ... I'd already done the sugar challenge and a few other detoxes but the Kick Start Fat Loss detox ... BAM! Body changed. Mindset changed. Confidence changed. I had a six pack. My body was ripped. These were massive changes.

I've always struggled with my weight. Throughout my life I've had yo-yo dieting issues, just eating what I thought was healthy ... believing any old thing I was told. As a busy instructor I looked fit but was always bloated, had a belly and back fat, plus I had bowel issues, eczema and always looked puffy in the face.

At my heaviest (in my 20s) I was 18 stone. I had gradually lost the weight but the Kick Start Fat Loss detox was the last part of the jigsaw. In the last two years, due to diet changes, I have lost two stone. The Kick Start Fat Loss way of eating totally works for me and makes a lot of sense. I have to eat to maintain my energy levels.

People soon started to notice my changes and my confidence. Don't get me wrong, I'm a born blagger, I appear confident, but I never really believed it myself. Since I started my journey with Kick Start Fat Loss all my other classes are now super busy. I have increased my profile.

This is so much more than I could have ever hoped for. When I started, I wanted everything now but now I see that it's a slow burner and you can work at your own pace. At the start I felt like I had to keep up but I understand now that you have to work at your pace.

I love the support, the sister hood and the positivity of Kick Start Fat Loss. It fits in perfectly with my lifestyle. I've always been a positive thinker, but now I'm part of a team of like minded, motivated people. Everyday is an opportunity to lead a tribe of wonderful women towards being the best they can be!

I have know doubt that my branch of Kick Start Fat Loss will grow and help so many people, but the beautiful thing is the growth in me as a woman and as a role model. Being part of Kick Start Fat Loss has helped me to be more confident in my business and as a leader.

For me, the biggest difference between Kick Start Fat Loss and other so called slimming clubs is the honesty. I look at the research of how to lose fat and it's clear that what we are doing is bang on point. I see the others as old and outdated. At Kick Start Fat Loss we are all fitness professionals with a huge amount of knowledge and experience and access to the latest nutrition and fitness information. We offer exercise and we deal with mind set and self esteem. Kick Start Fat Loss is the whole package.

Kick Start Fat Loss is about education and and helping people to become the healthiest, happiest person they can be. The more I learn, the more the whole programme makes more sense. The support is incredible. Each and every person in the group brings something unique and we are all committed to supporting each other and driving our message forward. Just do it! I love it.

Jackie Panks

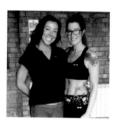

Mum of two, Jackie Panks (42) from Norfolk was determined to start her forties fit and fabulous. Having spent years dieting and attending various slimming clubs, Jackie was stuck in a rut feeling unfit, unmotivated and in need of a fresh approach to health and fitness. Jackie joined her local *Kick Start Fat Loss* with Jane Cole of The Fit Studios in Kings Lynn in 2013 and has since lost 21lbs and 26 inches.

I never did much exercise before joining Kick Start Fat Loss and it showed. I had low energy levels which left me feeling very lethargic.

Kick Start Fat Loss works on the principles of eliminating processed foods and empowering clients to achieve optimum well being through nutrition and fitness. I quickly felt the benefits since the plan taught me how to fuel my body properly in order to have more energy and maintain a healthy lifestyle.

As well as changing the way I ate, Kick Start Fat Loss helped me to develop a consistent fitness regime, which included running and HIIT (high intensity interval training) workouts. The workouts keep my body challenged and leave me energized, which I need as a busy mom of two, aged 10 and five.

I was once an emotional eater. Foods like chocolate and crisps were my staple diet. The ongoing support from Kick Start Fat Loss have given me the tools, knowledge and confidence to make positive food choices.

My typical diet before Kick Start Fat Loss was bran flakes and a banana for breakfast. Now it's turkey rashers, eggs and spinach.

Lunch before was a tuna sandwich, a low fat chocolate bar and crisps. Now it's a chicken and avocado salad.

Where previously I might eat a pasta bake with sauce from a jar and cheese for dinner, now it's salmon and sweet potato.

In twelve months I've lost a stone and a half and 26 inches of body fat.

My body has been transformed along with my attitude towards food, exercise and to me.

Kick Start Fat Loss has changed my life by giving me more energy with the children. I sleep better, and my skin and hair is healthier. I also have so much more body confidence now.

My advice to others is to try the plan for a month and see the difference in your body and mind. You will never look back.

Why Detox 1: Sugar Addiction

'I don't do sugar'

Let's start with sugar. One of the biggest barriers to fat loss is sugar addiction, something the initial detox aims to break.

The following questions are about your eating habits. Have a look through and answer them honestly.

Are you addicted to sugar?

1. Do you start the day with cereals and or toast?

2. When you find your energy slumps, do you crave carbohydrates or sugary snacks and food?

3. Do you crave sugary foods throughout the day.

4. Do you always have to include a 'sweet' dessert after you have a meal?

5. Do you eat more than 2/3 pieces of fruit per day?

6. If you cut out sugary foods do you experience withdrawal symptoms? For example: headaches, flu-like sniffles, generally bad mood/attitude?

7. Would you class your self as a chocoholic?

8. If you eat one biscuit/cake/chocolate/sweet can you not stop until you have eaten the whole packet and then crave more (even if you feel sick and bloated)?

9. Do you eat low fat or reduced fat foods?

10. Do you eat processed, tinned, microwaved or frozen foods regularly?

If you have answered yes to the majority of these questions (more than five) you are probably - along with a large percentage of the population - addicted to sugar.

Sugary processed foods trigger our brains to want more

You might think your craving for a biscuit or sweet bun is down to a lack of willpower but studies show that highly processed food is addictive in the same way as drugs like heroin or cocaine. A 2013 study, published in the American Journal of Clinical Nutrition, suggested that higher sugar, higher glycemic index foods can be addictive (Ludwig, 2013).[19] In other words, sugary processed foods trigger our brains to want more. It's not necessarily a lack of will power - it's an addiction.

David Ludwig (author of *Ending the Food Fight*), who led the Harvard study, found that foods that have a high glycemic index - which basically means foods that raise blood sugar more than table sugar (foods like white flour and refined starch) - trigger a region in the

---

[19] Ludwig. D (2013),*Effects of dietary glycemic index on brain regions related to reward and craving in men*, American Journal of Clinical Nutrition.

brain called the nucleus accumbens. This region is responsible for addictions, such as drug abuse.

There have been several studies which have shown this area of the brain lights up in response to sugary foods when compared to something less pleasurable, like a boiled vegetable but Ludwig's study goes further. It proves the connection between the biology of sugar, as in its glycaemic index and its affect on the brain, rather than just the appearance of something sweet and pleasurable to eat.

The fat trap
So if you consider that you might have a sugar addiction, could you then consider that your desire to find a diet which promises to enable you to lose weight whilst at the same time keeping these addictive foods firmly on the menu is part of the fat trap? Is this why super smart women who know this stuff still can't bring themselves to try anything but a calorie controlled diet because they just can't wean themselves off refined foods?

Hidden sugars
The scary part of all this is that you might not even think you are eating sugar. We often unwittingly consume hidden sugars added to foods we assume are 'healthy'. This is especially true of low fat foods where sugar is often used to make foods taste better.

If you're at home, go and take a look in your cupboards and your fridge now. Or next time you're at the shops, check out the label on a low fat fruit yoghurt. How high up the ingredients list is sugar?

Have you ever eaten a low fat yoghurt and craved more? Now imagine eating chicken and broccoli, it's unlikely you'd crave or have room for more chicken or broccoli than your body needs.

I really hope this is starting to ring some alarm bells with you. Before you start berating yourself for food choices which have kept you trapped in body fat, just stop. I'm trying to explain that so much of the fat trap is not actually your fault. At no point have I said to you, "you just need to eat less and move more," because if it were that simple YOU'D BE DOING IT!

You don't want to be fat. You don't want to eat rubbish. I know that. You know that. There are so many factors working against your good intentions. Poor advice; clever marketing and advertising campaigns that want you to think you are rubbish; and sugar!

Low fat ideology
We are in this trap because in the 1940s, scientists began to see a link between high fat diets and high cholesterol, suggesting that a low fat diet might prevent heart disease. In her article, *How the Ideology of Low Fat Conquered America*, Ann La Berge explains how the world (in particular the US) got carried away with the idea and by the 1980s low fat ideology prevailed (La Berge, 2008).[20] The ideology was promoted by doctors and governments (so we all believed it) but with little evidence to support the fact that low fat diets either prevented heart disease or helped weight loss. Americans were still getting fatter (along with the rest of the developed world).

---

[20] La Berge. A. F (2008) *How the Ideology of Low Fat Conquered America*, J Hist Med Allied Sci 63 (2): 139-177 first published online February 23, 2008doi:10.1093/jhmas/jrn001

We ignored sugar and the food industry got busy finding tasty alternatives to fat, which often meant adding sugar or sweeteners to give the food back the taste that taking the fat out took away!

Our shelves are full of additive and sugar laden food products
Roll on over thirty years and our shelves are full of additive and sugar laden food products. Entire diets are marketed on the idea of breakfast cereals and even baby or children's foods are highly processed.

Remember it's not just sugar that creates an addiction, it's highly processed, high glycaemic index foods. This includes potatoes, white pasta and white flour. It's everywhere.

When it comes to choosing what you eat, you have to become your own detective. One of my most successful participants, Lesley Gooch (who has now lost over nine stone having previously been a serial dieter), told me that the single biggest factor in changing her attitude and diet was understanding food marketing and food labels. Lesley has now become her own food detective. She can distinguish marketing hype from the truth. This is the only way to beat sugar addiction.

Fruit, fructose and 'healthy' sugars
Now you might be thinking, 'well that's okay - I can quit processed sugar because I can easily replace it with healthy sugars like fruit, honey and agave nectar.' You might think this but unfortunately for your taste buds, your body deals with refined sugars, fruit sugars and 'healthy' sugars all the same way. You might think you are going sugar free by swapping sugar for honey in your muffins but you are still feeding the sugar addiction and it's the sugar addiction we need to crack.

Any sugar entering the bloodstream is processed by the liver, which consequently switches on fat production and encourages laying down of fat cells around your mid section, that visceral fat which increases your risk of disease and gives you a gut!

Candida
It's not just your brain which could be triggering your desire for sweet food. It could be your gut too. It's easy to forget that our digestive system is a living, breathing organism that gives us feedback on our food choices.

We have bacteria living in our intestines which help us break down foods but which also feed off our food and like anything in our bodies, if we over do, or in this case over eat too much of one thing and neglect balance, our gut can get out of whack.

A detox can help restore our natural balance, which is also known as homeostasis, the point at which our body can function optimally.

One digestive gremlin is candida, a naturally occurring yeast or fungus (there are different strains so I'm generalising here). It lives in your intestines and mouth and helps with digestion and nutrient absorption. An overgrowth of candida (candidiasis) can trigger sweet cravings.

Scientists agree that candidiasis can be caused by a range of conditions such as a compromised immune system, stress, antibiotics, norovirus or high alcohol consumption. It is especially linked to diabetes and there is a definite link between raised blood sugar levels and increased candida levels.[21]

Too much refined food in your diet can increase your candida levels
Too much refined food in your diet can therefore increase your candida levels, it feeds the fungus. More fungus needs more sugar. Think of it like a forest of fungus multiplying inside your body. So whether an overgrowth has been caused by an uncontrollable factor or by high blood sugar levels (high stress plus high sugar consumption being a massive contributory factor) candida is quite possibly one of the leading charges in your sugar addiction.

Candidiasis can also lead to frequent yeast infections, bloating or loose stools, it can also be confused with gluten intolerance.

There is some evidence to suggest that too much candida can begin to break down the intestinal wall and penetrate the blood stream, leading to health problems. This is what's known as leaky gut. Leaky gut caused by candidiasis is still one of those conditions debated by the medical profession. It's thought leaky gut could be caused by certain drugs like aspirin or iboprofen, health conditions like coeliac disease, chemotherapy and HIV/AIDS but the sugar connection is less researched. Nutritional bodies like the Institute for Optimal Nutrition have however conducted research into candidiasis, yeast overgrowth and leaky gut and in his book *The Yeast Connection*, Dr William Crook deals at length with the sugar connection.

---

[21] http://www.ncbi.nlm.nih.gov/pmc/articles/PMC2855059/

My 'sugar trap' top ten

Sugar is an absolute minefield but the most important thing to remember is that it can alter your brain chemistry and mindset, sabotaging your good intentions. So here are my top ten best ways to escape the sugar trap:

1. **Don't add sugar to food or drinks.** The easiest way to immediately cut down on your sugar intake is to cut it out of tea and coffee.

2. **Don't be fooled by 'healthy' sugar.** Brown sugar, raw sugar or natural sugars like agave nectar are still sugar. Yes they are less refined but they act the same as sugar when they are ingested. Your body converts sugars and stores them as fat, almost as quickly as it would glucose.

3. **Reduce or eliminate processed carbohydrates.** Bread, biscuits and cake are just like sugar to the body too. A chocolate biscuit will just get stored as fat.

4. **Cut out fat free and low fat snacks.** It is a massive myth that a low fat label automatically makes that food healthy. Fat free does not mean calorie or sugar free. This is a tough myth to break but low fat foods will just keep you locked into your sugar addiction.

5. **Become a food detective.** In order to reduce sugar from your diet you need to know where it is. Start reading food labels. Here's a list of common 'hidden' sugars to get you started:

   - corn sweetener
   - corn syrup
   - dextrose
   - fructose
   - fruit juice concentrates
   - glucose
   - high-fructose corn syrup
   - invert sugar
   - lactose
   - maltose
   - malt syrup
   - raw sugar
   - sucrose
   - sugar syrup
   - cane crystals
   - cane sugar
   - crystalline fructose
   - evaporated cane juice
   - corn syrup solids
   - malt syrup

6. **Beware of artificial sweeteners.** Sweeteners and sugar replacements like Stevia can increase your cravings for sugar and some research suggests they could be more harmful to your body than sugar.

7. **Count your teaspoons.** Every 4g of sugar in a product is roughly the equivalent of a teaspoon. So count your grams of sugar and divide by four to find out how many teaspoons of sugar you are consuming.

8. **Limit your fruit intake.** Yes fruit does contain lots of fibre and healthy nutrients but so do vegetables. Fruit can be very high in sugar and your body can react to it in the same way as sugar. You don't need to give it up forever but whilst you're trying to lose fat and detox, fruit isn't your friend. Limit it to every other day and just low glycaemic index foods like berries and grapefruit after a workout.

9. **Eliminate fruit juice.** Fruit juice will just create a massive sugar hit and is really bad for your teeth too.

Why Detox 2: Gluten and Wheat Addiction

We all know that gluten isn't great for us but it's really hard to kick out from our diets.

There are two big reasons for this:

1. It's everywhere. In bread, in cakes, in processed foods like sauces and condiments, in crackers and cereals. The list goes on.

2. It's addictive. Consuming gluten affects our brain chemistry, like sugar and like drugs. We constantly crave more of it, in fact I'd even suggest that gluten could be one of the biggest things keeping our nation fat!

Why?

Gluten is highly addictive
Like sugar, gluten is highly addictive. It leaves us craving more.

Your body reacts to wheat and gluten with a big blood sugar spike. And if your blood sugar levels increase, so will your blood insulin levels.

Too much sugar and insulin over time can lead to insulin resistance, which in turn leads to laying down fat around your tummy. Otherwise known as a wheat belly!

It's relatively easy to spot the way your body reacts to gluten and wheat in your system too since the whole process takes around two hours.

So let's say you start the day with your favourite whole wheat cereal or a couple of slices of whole grain toast. You feel satisfied. However, your toast is the equivalent to four teaspoons of sugar and a bowl of breakfast cereal, even those marketed as healthy, may contain the equivalent of up to six teaspoons of sugar.

Your body reacts to your breakfast with that big blood sugar high. This triggers the insulin response. Then two hours later you are hungry again - usually craving more wheat or sugary foods.

Gluten, wheat and inflammation
Gluten is hugely inflammatory. The minute you take it out of your diet you'll notice a big difference around your gut and your mid section.

If you suffer with inflammatory conditions such as arthritis, eczema or bowel conditions like IBS, cutting out gluten from your diet can minimize your symptoms within days.

Your body can become inflamed if it's been under assault from toxins or stress
Inflammation is your body's way of protecting itself. In the same way as your ankle may swell if you have tripped and sprained it, your body can become inflamed if it's been under assault from toxins or stress.

Unfortunately we tend to ignore inflammation when it isn't from a fall. So you might wake with a puffy face or joints or perhaps with a strange headache and put it down to 'one of those things,' but it is often as a result of something you've eaten that hasn't agreed with you. And if you ignore your body, over time, this inflammation can become chronic.

This is why, when you start the *Kick Start Fat Loss* programme we have a detox to kick out all known allergens and irritants.

Modern wheat and Super Gluten
Move over Superman, super gluten is coming to town. Wheat today is very different to what we might have eaten 50 or 60 years ago.

On a practical level, we no longer have a mill round the corner with a local miller grinding grain from his farm. Farming methods have changed radically.

Increased consumer demand, mass production and changes in farming will all have affected the quality of wheat we consume and the treatment of the original grain.

Some researchers have even suggested that as a result of production and farming changes there is now such a thing as super gluten, which is even more inflammatory and addictive than regular old gluten.

As with all foods, it's important to be your own food detective. Look for foods which are close to their original farm source and as near to unprocessed as possible. If you don't know what's in your food, then at least for the duration of your time with *Kick Start Fat Loss*, kick it out.

Cutting out gluten - the come down
The biggest challenge with cutting out gluten, aside from finding good alternatives to bread and pasta, is that you'll get some withdrawal symptoms. When your brain is craving more you could feel pretty ropey. Just keep focusing on the positive changes your dietary changes will have on your health.

Your brain health and function and your waist line will feel a massive difference and you won't crave sugar or wheat-based foods so frequently.

Once you come out of the other side of your food withdrawal you will feel great and you will notice it. This isn't just about dropping body fat. Yes that will happen. But this is about how you will mentally feel. How you'll feel sharper and more energised.

Kick Start Fat Loss focuses on your mental and brain performance too
This is something I feel has been missing from so many diet plans over the years. We've tended to focus on how you look and what dress size you are or you want to be. *Kick Start Fat Loss* focuses on your mental and brain performance too. Those times when you can't remember a word, a name or a place. You get brain fog too. Once you take all of those inflammatory and irritant foods away you'll start to feel amazing. The pleasure is absolutely worth the pain!

Reactions to foods might not be instant
Don't forget as well that reactions to foods might not be instant. You might eat some pasta on a Monday but not start to get joint pain or bloating for a few days. It doesn't mean it isn't the food that's causing the reaction, it can just be delayed. This is why keeping a food log or a food diary can really help you when it comes to understanding how you react to foods and how foods can affect your moods and mental clarity.

Skip the 'free-from' ranges
It is important to remember that if you're planning on cutting out gluten, I'd advise strongly against replacing the foods you've 'lost' with foods from the 'free from' ranges in supermarkets. Like any processed foods, 'free from' foods can contain sugars and additives and just like any food buying, you'll need to be your own food detective in order to ensure what you're putting in your trolley and subsequently your body is not going to hinder your progress.

Why Detox 3: Dairy

"My entire family is now 'dairy free'. I've tried to re-introduce small amounts back into my diet but as soon as I do I get a blocked nose and sinuses. I lived for entire winters with sinusitis before I realised it was a dairy intolerance."

[Fiona McMeechan, Essex]

We all believe dairy has to be good for us. It's the typical wholesome drink for children or pregnant women. Full of calcium to make growing bones strong.

Babies are nurtured on it.
There are endless campaigns marketing yoghurts and 'pro-gut health' milky drinks as a nutritional 'cure-all.'

Do you believe the hype?
"Well I just felt rubbish every day until I started my daily yoghurt eating ritual, whilst languishing on a velvet sofa. Now I just bounce out of bed in the morning, with barely the need for make up and when I poo it's like butterflies come out of my bottom!" [Said Nobody, Ever]

Let's get a little more Diet Detective about this. According to a 2012 study on the evolution of lactase persistence the majority of adults have at least some difficulty in digesting milk (Leonardi, Gerbault, Thomas and Berger, 2012)[22].

The article found that whilst most young children produce lactase and can digest the lactose in their mother's milk, as they mature, most switch off the lactase gene. Only 35% of the human population can digest lactose beyond the age of about seven or eight.

Do you like milk?
How do you feel after you've eaten foods like double cream or cheese cake?

Before I share the facts on why we avoid dairy on the *Kick Start Fat Loss* detox, it's worth thinking for yourself about how these foods make you feel.

Why do we avoid dairy on the *Kick Start Fat Loss* detox?

Pasteurization
One of the main problems with cow's milk in our diets is the process of pasteurization. Milk is pasteurized to control harmful microbes and to help preserve it. These days few off us have easy access to a local dairy farm.

During the pasteurization process, milk is heated to 150 degrees fahrenheit for 30 minutes before it is stored at temperatures below 55 degrees fahrenheit. As well as the positives, this heating process kills off beneficial probiotics in the milk, and changes the structure of milk proteins (denatures milk proteins), transforming the raw milk to a product which can sit on the supermarket shelves for our convenience.

Of course, with any processing, there are some nutritional losses.

Downsides of pasteurization
Pasteurization turns milk lactose sugars into beto lactose sugars that the body absorbs faster. Sugars that are absorbed faster will create the sugar spikes which happen after eating refined foods.

It's also worth remembering that humankind existed and drank milk long before Louis Pasteur made his famous discovery.

What is Casein?

Casein represents 80 percent of the protein in cow's milk. As well as being drunk and used in cheese production, casein is used for making plastics, glue and paint!

For the purposes of the *Kick Start Fat Loss* detox, casein is hard to digest.

[22] Leonard. M, Gerbault. P, Thomas. M and Burger. J (2011), *The evolution of lactase persistence in Europe. A synthesis of archaeological and genetic evidence*, International Dairy Journal, Volume: 22 Issue: 2 Pages: 88-9 DOI: 10.1016/j.idairyj.2011.10.010 Published: FEB 2012

Cow's milk is very different to breast milk. The fact that cows have four stomachs and humans just the one, gives us a clue that we may not have the best equipment for digesting cow's milk.

Casein forms dense curds in the stomach, great for filling us up, but not so easy for all of us to digest.

One of the focuses of the *Kick Start Fat Loss* detox is getting our digestive health into the best state possible to aid fat loss and make us feel great. Any food group that makes digestion or our bodies work harder isn't going to serve our detox purposes.

What about calcium?
Milk has typically been marketed as a great source of calcium (although some evidence suggests pasteurization transforms the calcium in milk so the human body cannot easily absorb it).

So cutting it out of our diets might leave you concerned that you'll be putting yourself at risk of conditions like osteoporosis or brittle bones.

You don't need dairy for calcium
Green vegetables like kale, spinach and broccoli contain massive amounts of calcium along with loads of other vitamins and minerals.

Load bearing exercise
During *Kick Start Fat Loss* you'll be doing plenty of exercise to help minimise your risk of osteoporosis.

You don't need dairy for vitamin D
Yes, milk is fortified with vitamin D but actually only about a fifth of your daily requirement. Sun is the number one source of vitamin D since we can easily absorb it but eggs, meat and fish are all great sources too.

Why Detox 4: Alcohol

Sadly I am not about to give you a clean alcohol consumption plan.

There is no such thing as healthy alcohol.

Yes. Some types of alcohol are lower in sugar and additives than others but all alcohol consumption leads to:

• Food cravings;
• Brain fog; and of course
• Loss of willpower.

While you are detoxing try not to drink alcohol at all.

Your drinking days aren't completely over
When the detox is complete and you're in the maintenance phase of *Kick Start Fat Loss* then there are some guidelines for drinking alcohol.

But for now, be honest about the way alcohol affects your mental function and health.

Alcohol stops your body burning fat
When you drink alcohol you stop burning fat. Your liver sees alcohol as a poisonous substance and works hard to process and remove it. So all fat burning is switched off while the liver deals with alcohol.

The way your body processes foods is complex. It needs to convert foods into energy. If we throw alcohol into the mix all those processes are put on hold in order to eliminate this toxin.

This means fat is not oxidised (you stop burning fat), it becomes much easier for your body to lay down dietary fat and you don't absorb nutrients from food as you did when you were sober.

In a nutshell, if you want to maintain a lean body, avoiding alcohol is a good choice.

It's not just the added calories (alcohol has seven calories per gram compared to carbohydrates and protein, which contain four each), alcohol affects metabolism because when you drink it, your body puts all other metabolic processes on hold until it has processed the alcohol.

Your body can't convert the calories from alcohol to fat, meaning it needs to use them up, and will delay all other fat burning and energy use until the alcohol has been processed.

Drinking alcohol affects your hormones as well, increasing cortisol and modifying steroid metabolism in the liver. This results in lower androgens for both sexes. Women with higher levels of androgens and men with lower levels are equally at risk for belly fat gain, and for men, lower androgens mean less testosterone.

Drinking alcohol also increases your cortisol levels, which makes those sugar spikes worse. And by increasing your sugar consumption you will crave carbohydrates the next day.

But what of those parties?
I can't ask you to stop drinking forever. There is a balance to life after all.

Once you have finished your detox and you're ready to maintain your goals, here are some strategies to help you through your party.

1. Make the night of the party your cheat meal. Drink whatever you want but accept that the following day you will have the hangover from hell. You'll crave sugar and carbs and feel pretty low. Can you deal with that?

2. Vodka and gin have the lowest sugar content. Add a soda water and a splash of lemon or lime juice.

3. Champagne and sparkling white wines are better for you than red wine or beers.

4. Beer contains toxins and grains. If you drink beer on a regular basis you are unlikely to lose weight.

5. On the day of your party eat a protein rich breakfast, lunch and dinner.

6. Drink green tea through the day before you drink alcohol.

7. Take your usual supplements.

8. Eat a protein rich breakfast the following day to minimize carb and sugar cravings.

Does this make drinking okay?

Not really.

Theoretically, you could be looking at four or more ounces of alcohol in a typical 'social' evening, clocking in at a likely total of somewhere between 256 to 328 calories (and I'm being conservative).

Your body can't store alcohol, so it has to use it up first. Remember all other metabolic processes, like metabolizing fat and glucose have to be put on hold while your body gets rid of the alcohol.

The occasional drink wont sabotage your fat loss just ensure you eat your protein rich meals before and after.

Beware of Drinking after Detox
After you have completed the *Kick Start Fat Loss* I wouldn't encourage you to drink a lot all at once.

Your body is clean and will treat the alcohol as a poison, potentially making you vomit or worse!

Go easy and tread carefully. Remember alcohol makes you lose your inhibitions and you might not need much encouraging to head for your favourite munchies.

What *Kick Start Fat Loss* participant have said about the detox

I asked some of my *Kick Start Fat Loss* participants around the country to share their thoughts on the *Kick Start Fat Loss* detox. This is what they said:

"Since doing the Kick Start Fat Loss detox, I've kicked my caffeine addiction. I feel energised, stronger, and my premenstrual dysphoric disorder (PMDD) this month is non-existent (usually I am chopping heads off at this point in my cycle). There's some definition in my muscles, and the biggest tell of all - I can finally fit my wedding band back on my finger without it cutting off the circulation! Brilliant!"

[Sophie, 25]

"Before I started the Kick Start Fat Loss detox I was getting regular hot flushes during the night which were keeping me awake. Since the detox I have had no flushes whatsoever and am sleeping batter than I have done in years. Weight and inch loss is an added bonus especially when I feel so full all the time."

[Andrea Riddoch, 47, Leeds]

"The Kick Start Fat Loss programme has delivered on weight and inch loss but most detoxes will do that. What makes this programme outstanding is the education, support and motivation that I know will have a long lasting impact on my health and well being."

[Jayne Hume, 37, Birmingham]

"If you are serious about losing weight getting stronger and happier then Kick Start Fat Loss is for you! After only 7 days on the Kick Start Fat Loss detox, my energy levels were up, my mood lifted and yes, I felt a lot lighter! Kick Start Fat Loss fits into your everyday life ... It's not gimmicky and not calorie counting. It's A WAY OF LIFE!"

[Natalie Hill, Gibraltar, 31]

"Seven days of the Kick Start Fat Loss detox and I have shed the 8lbs that I'd been struggling to lose for years! I feel awesome on this plan. Sharp minded, energised and empowered. This is the future of healthy eating!"

[Claire Tonkin, Surrey, 35]

"Since being on Kick Start Fat Loss I haven't had my usual monthly hormonal 'ups and downs' and my nightly hot sweats have totally vanished! Kick Start Fat Loss is a healthy diet for life as well as the added bonus of losing weight too. Join the Revolution!"

[Arlene Woodward, Sheffield, 47]

"In 7 days I lost 6lbs after months of not dropping weight. I feel fab. No bloated tummy and loads of energy."

[Suzanne Richardson, Dudley, 36]

"Since doing the upgraded Kick Start Fat Loss detox, I have realised that I don't have to keep snacking on 'healthy foods' to keep me going. I now eat two or three meals instead. I have so much more energy to do the things I keep putting off. I think clearer all day and sleep better. I feel very positive about my body, as I can see it changing daily. I know this will not be just a detox, Kick Start Fat Loss will be a lifestyle change."

[Sara Calder, 28]

"After seven days on Kick Start Fat Loss I lost 8lbs. My PMT and period was hugely different. I suffer with fibroids so it was a huge step forwards. My sleep is fabulous and I'm up with a spring in my step. I suffer with sarcoidosis which can be painful. Clean eating has given me more energy and I feel rebalanced all over again."

[Joanne Roome, 41]

Chris Tuck

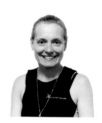

Chris has been a *Kick Start Fat Loss* franchise holder since 2012. She is based in West Wickham. Chris was already a fitness and health instructor but had struggled herself with eating disorders and chronic health conditions. Chris found the clean eating programme helped to keep her physically and mentally on track and she loves the authenticity and nutritional content of *Kick Start Fat Loss*. Chris is 44 and lives in West Wickham.

"For me, eating clean isn't about weight. It's about my physical and mental health. I use clean eating to keep my osteoarthritis and pain under control but I also need it because I have a history of eating disorders and still, when I'm under stress, I struggle with bulimia.

"Clean eating helps me stay on track. I'll be eating clean and then I get a trigger. Usually related to being abused as a child. I love a chocolate bar but if I eat one because of the trigger or because I'm stressed, I think, "I shouldn't be doing that," then the guilt kicks in and I make myself sick.

"Over Easter I found myself eating lots of chocolate. I was stressed. I had a lot going on with work and I was getting frustrated. There was chocolate around and for a couple of days I let myself wallow. But then I thought, "I know better." A lot of people get into a cycle of eating and can't get out of it.

"Emotional eating is a massive issue. I've noticed over the last two to three years of leading Kick Start Fat Loss groups that clients don't fall off because they don't want to see the end result, they fall off because of stress. So now we work on strategies to help stay on track. Strategies I've developed through my own issues with food.

"As a Kick Start Fat Loss instructor being able to talk about my own issues with my clients really helps everyone. When they first come they look at me and must think, "she's skinny, what does she know?" I tell them what I've been through and about my relationship with food. I just think they'll either walk because of what I tell them or they'll work with me.

"Treat foods should be exactly that, a treat and not a crutch. If I eat a chocolate bar it needs to be because I want it and because I'm happy to treat myself not because of a trigger.

"So when it comes to treats we have to ask ourselves, "why is it I want it and do I want to enjoy it?"

"Clean eating habits are so engrained in my psyche now that I know if I go on a cycle of bad eating I'll end up back to my bulimic habits. If I start to eat unhealthy stuff I ask myself why am I doing it.

"We need to know the difference between gut hunger and emotional hunger. Are you feeding an emotion?

"I'm pretty blunt with my clients. I tell them you've got enough fat on your body to fuel you. If you keep feeding yourself it's never going to come off.

I still have problems with fasting. I was starved and often hungry as a child so I need to have a full belly. If I start to fast and my tummy is empty, alarm bells go off in my head and then it's just eat eat eat.

I'd originally started doing a lot of nutritional research back in 2010 because of problems I'd been having with my hips. In the two years prior to having hip surgery to remove bone spurs, noone had ever mentioned nutrition and the part it could play in osteoarthritis. I wanted to look into holistic solutions for my osteoarthritis so I started Googling osteoarthritis and nutrition kept coming up.

My research and the information I learned from courses I attended all pointed to the fact that lots of what I was eating was inflammatory for my hips. I went from eating a predominantly low fat, low sugar diet with lots of pasta to protein, no processed foods and loads of vegetables.

I now understand the importance of vegetables in my diet. Before, I was just so busy that vegetables weren't on my radar. I couldn't be bothered to cook them. I just ate fruit. Tons of fruit, which I now know was creating a really acidic state in my body which is really bad for any inflammation, like osteoarthritis.

By changing the way I eat, my osteoarthritis is under control. It hasn't got worse. I'm managing it now. Vegetables are now my main priority.

All the research I'd done meant that when I found out about Rachel's Kick Start Fat Loss system I already knew this worked. So it was easy to jump on board. I believed in the programme.

I knew about Rachel and knew that with her knowledge and expertise the programme would be brilliant.

And it is. The Kick Start Fat Loss programme is great. It's not just a club. It's an online programme with support from a leader like me and the nutrition and exercise is what all the experts are preaching about at the moment.

Clean eating is not a passing phase it's my life."

Lisa Lockwood

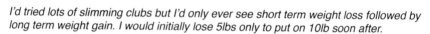

44-year-old Lisa Lockwood from Lowestoft, started *Kick Start Fat Loss* at Fen Park Primary School in January 2015. Lisa lost 15 pounds in the first month of *Kick Start Fat Loss* and has gone on to lose over four and a half stones in total.

Before Kick Start Fat Loss I had been a typical yo-yo dieter. But years of crash dieting and restrictive calorie counting had taken their toll on my metabolism. I felt hungry all the time and never got the results I wanted from dieting.

I'd tried lots of slimming clubs but I'd only ever see short term weight loss followed by long term weight gain. I would initially lose 5lbs only to put on 10lb soon after.

I suffered from chronic fatigue and joint aches after only standing for a few minutes. As a hair dresser and mum of three life became exhausting.

In the end I felt so frustrated I sought medical advice from my GP. Blood tests revealed I was suffering from an under active thyroid – a condition in which there is a reduced level of thyroid hormone (thyroxine) in the body. Common symptoms included tiredness, weight gain, constipation, aches, dry skin and feeling cold. Rather than feeling relieved to finally know what was wrong, I just resigned myself to being fat forever.

I had zero energy and no enthusiasm.

My wedding ring no longer fitted. I didn't believe that I could lose weight so ate more in comfort.

The turning point came on New Year's Eve 2014 – the annual family party. After looking forward to dressing as Cinderella, I was devastated when the size 18 dress did not fit.

Tipping the scales at 14st 7lbs and emotionally at an all time low, I knew it was time for change.

I was so tired of dreaming about being thinner.

On 5th January 2015, I joined Kick Start Fat loss club Lowestoft – ran by franchisee Helen Pybus. The Kick Start Fat Loss is a long term life style plan that works on the principles of clean eating and freshly prepared home cooked meals. There is no calorie counting or low fat foods – instead the emphasis is on eliminating sugar and eating as close to nature as possible.

In three weeks I lost an amazing 15 lbs!

The first few days were tough as I had scrapped sugar from my diet and my body soon realized this.

I'd always thought that I had eaten pretty healthily but Kick Start Fat Loss taught me so much about nutrition and the many foods out there that you think are healthy yet contain hidden sugars.

In just five months I lost 3 stone and I'm well on my way to losing the last 14lbs to get me to my goal weight.

This is the most amount of weight I have ever lost in this time frame and I definitely do not feel like I'm on a faddy diet.

With the help of the Kick Start Fat Loss Recipe Book I'm creating healthy and mouth watering meals that all my family are enjoying.

My confidence and self esteem have gone through the roof. A few days ago I got into a size 12 skirt. It felt so good.

My clothes are too big and I've had to have my wedding ring made smaller.

The aches, pains and tiredness I used to experience from my underactive thyroid have improved so much just from changing my diet. I used to feel awful every day. Now it's very very rarely. Normally only if I've had a late night.

I don't think I could have achieved this much without the support from my instructor and franchisee Helen Pybus. Helen is full of energy, passion, knowledge and kindness. Kick Start Fat Loss has changed the way I think about food and I am healthier and happier for it.

My advice for anyone who is struggling to lose weight and keep it off:

1. *Join a Kick Start Fat Loss group – you will learn so much about the food you eat and how it nourishes your body.*

2. *Don't beat yourself up if you have a bad day. It happens to us all. Just how eating clean for one day won't make you slimmer, eating badly on one day won't make you fat either.*

3. *Prepare your food in advance. This will ensure you are not tempted to make a detour and eat junk food.*

4. *Don't give up. Everyone deserves to lead a fulfilled and happy life. Kick Start Fat Loss will help you get there."*

Carlie Goode

47-year-old Carlie Goode's story is a little different from the big fat loss stories you might expect of a diet and lifestyle programme. Carlie started *Kick Start Fat Loss* in Banbury in September 2014 when her M.E. had begun to take over her life. Carlie still can't make the exercise sessions but the changes she's made to her diet have already changed her life. Carlie is testimony to the power of social media and that *Kick Start Fat Loss* can work remotely as well as in person.

Here's Carlie's inspiring story:

I've always believed that in life everything happens for a reason and that people are placed in our pathways at times through life when we need it most.

I was just scrolling down Facebook one day feeling really rubbish about myself, how I looked and where my life was at and happened to see something Kick Start Fat Loss had posted. I messaged Sindy to ask if she could help me with nutrition and losing weight given my circumstances. I had M.E. and could do zero exercise. Sindy came to meet me in September 2014.

I'd spent many years yo yo dieting. When I met Sindy I was the heaviest I had ever been at 12 stone 13. When I met Sindy I instantly felt a huge sense of how much she wanted to help me and how much she genuinely cared about my situation.

I was suffering from a debilitating condition which meant I couldn't do any of her classes. At the time I spent the majority of my day in bed, sleeping! The extent of physical activity for me was walking around my ground floor flat doing the minimal daily tasks with lengthy rests or sleep in between. I spent most of my time either sitting or lying down. In spite of this, Sindy was confident that not only could Kick Start Fat Loss help me lose weight but also have a positive impact on my health condition.

In 2006 I was diagnosed with M.E. also known as chronic fatigue syndrome. I'd experienced some symptoms many years before but it was in 2006, after the birth of my daughter, that it really hit and began to massively affect my life.

M.E. is hard to explain, even the medical profession are a little flummoxed as to what causes it, which means there is no treatment. I would describe M.E. as a set of symptoms that include fatigue, muscle pain, muscle weakness, headaches, blurred vision, foggy brain and lack of concentration.

Chronic fatigue is very different to feeling tired all the time. Chronic fatigue is like having the flu, after having had a heavy night out drinking, having run 10 miles and then physically, mentally and emotionally not being able to move! Showering, washing your hair, washing up, the minimal tasks become something you have to fight to do and some days are impossible.

For all the years I've suffered, I've found it impossible to describe to people exactly how it feels and the impact it has on your life.

To help explain, here's an example of a 'good' day in my life with M.E.:

I wake up and get my daughter to school.
I come home and sleep until it's time to pick her up.

I get her dinner sorted.

I get her to bed.

Then I go back to bed myself.

That's it!

When I started my journey with Kick Start Fat Loss I was not in a good place. I hated what I looked like. I was depressed and felt like life was just passing me by. I was existing not living.

When I first joined Kick Start Fat Loss I was unable to attend meetings but Sindy visited weekly to weigh me and give me advice. I was also part of the online group.

I am a fussy eater and to be honest, I don't like vegetables so at first I thought, 'I am not going to be able to do this!' I haven't been 'on it' religiously - no one is perfect and I think we all fall off the wagon from time to time - but for me juicing has been a godsend! My favourite at the moment is carrot, apple, banana and blueberry! I also found I could have vegetables too by adding them to the juice and not even tasting them.

The changes in my body have kept me motivated. I'm getting back into clothes I never dreamt I would wear again.

Sindy's attitude, support and guidance have also been a massive help along with the Facebook group. Seeing how everyone is doing and how supportive everyone is of each other is inspiring. I hope that soon I'll be able to start coming to meetings to meet people in the group.

So how do I feel now? I like myself again. I'd still like to lose more weight but I no longer look in the mirror and think I look vile. I can look in the mirror and feel proud of what I've achieved. I like the way I look.

I am now 11 stone 2 but have lost a lot of inches and am now back in size 12 jeans that I haven't worn for eight years. I've achieved this with very little exercise. I'm not promoting inactivity, if I could then I would. If I can achieve this then I believe every single person out there can. If there are some days you don't manage to exercise, don't beat yourself up. You can still achieve big results.

Thank you to Sindy and every one who is a member of Kick Start Fat Loss for the posts you all put up.

Dream. Believe. Achieve!

Frequently Asked Questions

We are very nearly there. Soon you'll be ready to start the detox and kick start your fat loss. But before we do there are a few frequently asked questions (and answers) to ensure the last of your queries are resolved.

It's only natural to have questions, so here are some of those most commonly asked:

Why do I have to moderate my fruit intake?
Fruit contains sugar and, although it is a natural sugar, the body reacts to it in the same way as regular sugar. If you must eat fruit stick to a few pieces every other day and only low GI fruits like water melon, grapefruit or berries after a workout.

Will I have to make separate meals for my family?
NO! We really hope your family will get behind you and support you all the way. Get everyone involved and interested in clean eating. This is a lifestyle change and one we hope you will continue with into the future. There is no evidence to suggest children need to eat processed foods, we've just got used to it. Children thrive on home cooked food too.

I haven't got time to cook and I'm not that great at cooking anyway!
Don't worry. All the meals and recipe ideas can be made in a matter of minutes. You really don't have to be a chef to enjoy cooking from scratch with good quality ingredients. Get a slow cooker so you always have a ready meal and plan in advance.

Which cooking methods can I use?
We would recommend steaming, stir frying, oven baking, grilling and using a slow cooker.

What happens when I go back to eating 'normally'?
We would advise you to continue following the *Kick Start Fat Loss* plan, using the 'treat meal' method. If you return to your old eating habits, you will experience the same results those eating habits gave you.

Isn't it dangerous to eat more than three eggs per week, will I increase my cholesterol?
No, it isn't dangerous. There are two types of cholesterol, 'good' and 'bad' known as HDL and LDL respectively. Eggs contain good cholesterol and are fine to be included regularly in your diet. In fact a 2012 study revealed that eggs can also keep you fuller for longer if you eat them at breakfast time (Dhurandhar, 2012).[23] Researchers from the Louisiana State University compared egg eating with cereal eating where both had the same amount of protein and the eggs still won.

Why can't I eat things that are from a gluten free range, like bread, cookies etc?
Be cautious of assuming something 'gluten free' is healthy. It's still a processed food and can therefore still contain hidden sugars or preservatives.

Where will I get my energy from if I cut my carbohydrates?
Carbohydrates are not limited to bread, pasta and potatoes, they are found in all fruit and vegetables.

---

[23] Dhurandhar, NV. '*Breakfast containing egg proteins induces greater satiety compared to a breakfast with lower protein quality.*' European Congress on Obesity 2012. Lyon, France. May 12, 2012.

So you won't be cutting carbohydrates out from your diet, you will be limiting 'starchy' carbs but eating loads of energy rich carbs like green vegetables.

Doesn't bread help regulate your bowel movements?
NO! In fact, it can do the exact opposite. Modern wheat is very heavily processed and can aggravate the gut wall. Some people find bread products very difficult to digest and it's another processed food with hidden sugars and starchy carbs that you don't need.

Isn't wholemeal/rye/dark/brown/granary etc bread is good for you?
These products will also contain gluten, are very carb-heavy and stress the digestive system.

Isn't drinking too much water dangerous?
We recommend you drink three litres of water per day to help eliminate excess toxins from your body and hydrate your cells. A hydrated body is a more efficient engine and if you're working out more you'll need to replenish fluid and drink to help muscle recovery.

Can I flavour my water with cordial?
No. Some cordials contain a sugar substitute called aspartame; an intense sweetener, around 200 times sweeter than sugar. Others contain sugar. Stick to water.

Isn't red wine good for you?
No. It contains sugar. Regardless of any antioxidants in red wine, the body will react to as if it's sugar. Also consider how many times you may have made a poor food choice following alcohol consumption. When you drink alcohol, your liver stops metabolising fat and concentrates on dealing with breaking down the alcohol so, in effect, when you drink your body stops processing fat.

I'm at a party in two weeks time, what is the best alcoholic drink to have?
Unfortunately, there isn't one. All alcohol has the same effect. If you want results, then you have to make changes!

What can I use as stock?
You can use the juices from cooked meat and add fresh or dried herbs. Try pouring it into ice cube trays and freezing them for future use.

Can I have decaf coffee?
No. In order to remove caffeine, the coffee beans must go through a process which often involves chemicals. In addition to this, to be classified as decaf, the product only needs to contain 97% less caffeine than traditional coffee.

If I already attend fitness classes and/or go to the gym, can I continue to do so?
Yes. However, the *Kick Start Fat Loss* workouts must come first as they are designed to work with the diet plan.

Do I have to have a rest day?
Yes. Your body needs time to repair and rebuild. We would recommend at least 1 rest day per week.

How important is it to stick to the nutrition plan?
Crucial. Your nutrition forms around 80% of your results. Exercise will speed up the process and supplements do exactly what their name suggests; supplement a great nutrition and exercise plan.

I'm premenstrual and have powerful cravings.
Your *Kick Start Fat Loss* leader will suggest ideas for cravings. Keep drinking lots of water and stay busy, cravings are more often than not in the mind.

Kick Start Fat Loss is for 28 days. That's only 28 days out of your life. I promise that you will see amazing results; your body shape will change, you will have so much more energy and feel alive and vital.

I'm Vegetarian will the plan be suitable for me?
Yes of course, your leader will be able to assist you with your vegetarian options. Stick with the plan 100% and it will change your life forever.

I would like more recipe and meal ideas!
Visit www.KickStartFatLoss.net and log into the members' area to find your additional workouts and recipe ideas.

Kick Start Fat Loss: The programme

So here we are. You know the facts. You know the science. You even know that your shopping lists and cooking habits are about to radically change. But before we launch into your cupboard re-organisation. It is vital to prepare your mind.

This is where *Kick Start Fat Loss* is different and this is why it really works. We start with education, continue with mindset and finish with great results that you'll want to share.

You could start on your detox now (no one is going to tell you not to) but I'd encourage you to take a moment to read the next few pages about mindset and to really take some time out to set goals for yourself, since this preparation is what's going to see you through to your goal.

Mindset and goal setting

Today I'm going to challenge you to make up your mind to live life differently.

Of course, you've tried this before and it probably hasn't worked (that's why you're reading this book) but I have some tips that really work. They've worked for all the women I've shared them with who now have the physique they have always dreamed of or the business they have always wanted.

What are they?

1. Become a 21st century list maker.

2. Decide what you want to achieve.

3. Coping with falling off the wagon and contingency planning

Become a 21st century list maker

If you're going to do one thing differently after you've read this book or make one change today, I'd encourage you to change the way you make lists.

Having clear goals and a positive mindset on top of the right knowledge is what's going to get you to your goals. And please forgive me, I know this all sounds obvious but I have a few tricks to share to transform your lists from a dog eared, sticky 'to do' note on your fridge (that stays there whilst you're out at work all day) to a twenty first century 'done it' list.

You may already be a list maker. You may not. But listen up. This next bit is important.

Make your list a place where your lifestyle goals sit alongside your everyday tasks
I'm not just talking about shopping, jobs or food here. I want you to make your list a place where your lifestyle goals sit alongside your everyday tasks. We are putting everything together on this. It's time to move forwards with your mental wellbeing. Beating yourself up because of a setback will not serve you long term. If your motivation starts to take a nose

dive and your aspirations and positivity are stuck inside your posh notebook in the depths of your designer handbag, whilst you dive into the nearest sweet shop, then I'd suggest that your list isn't working for you.

Goal setting, time management and mindset are all subjects I've read extensively about. I love to sit with a special pencil and map out my day and I still do write it all down but then I transfer it onto my smart phone. We check our phones a lot. Even if you aren't into social media, I'm sure you check your phone more than your posh notebook.

I love the iPhone reminders app. You may already be using it. But now it's time to add your lifestyle goals onto your list making.

Write a list
So here's the first step. Grab a piece of paper (or your favourite notebook) and write a list. We'll go into a bit more detail on goal setting later but for now, I'd encourage you to write your list for today (or if it's late it can be for tomorrow). Five things you want to get done today.

Re-evaluate your list
Let's say you've got to the end of the day and your list is feeling abandoned. You haven't fired through your tasks with your usual gusto.

What do you do now?

• Be realistic. It's okay. We all have days when we're full of energy and we're super productive but not every day is like that. Go with your energy. Work from your master list and be honest about what you are likely to achieve on any particular day.

• Be honest. Did you deliberately put something off or was it beyond your control? Yes be realistic but there are times where you'll need to push through a little bit.

• Sleep on it. Things are often easier to process after a break. Go back to your list fresh and ask yourself if the tasks are still important. Re-prioritize.

• Be flexible. Your list is there to guide you towards your goals, not to make you feel like a failure.

Decide what you want to achieve: Goal Setting

Here's how we set our goals at *Kick Start Fat Loss*. Our goals are those aims we have for our fat loss, our physical appearance and our mental wellbeing. Remember *Kick Start Fat Loss* is not just about transforming your shape. It's about your performance, your mental clarity and your happiness too. So think big. Grab your piece of paper and a quiet place and get your goals down.

Goal setting check list

1. Write your goals down and be descriptive and clear

2. Consider your goals by completing the following sentences:

- My perfect weight is ...
- My body will look like ... (describe your ideal shape, muscle tone etc)
- My energy levels are ...
- My mind set is ...

3. Next write down everything you hope to get out of this program.

If you would like to share these goals on the *Kick Start Fat Loss* Facebook page please do.

I really hope that you are starting to feel excited and elated knowing you are going to achieve your dreams and you can turn your goals into reality.

Falling off the wagon and contingency planning

EVERYONE will fall off the clean eating, healthy lifestyle bandwagon. Our eating habits aren't called 'habits' for nothing. One of the main reasons for doing a 28 day detox is to try to break those habits - but that's not to say it will be easy.

It is important to state from the beginning that slip ups are an inevitable part of the process. Yes, you might feel full of vigor and motivation on day one but part of success is contingency planning. Preparing yourself for when temptation strikes or giving up feels like an easier and safer option.

It is okay to fall off the wagon. It is normal to be tempted and at times to give in to that temptation but how can we ensure that you jump right back on again?

Get back on the wagon and stay on it
I've found that the men and women who are most successful, are those who get back on the wagon and stay on it. Those that falter are those who keep jumping off and on again - eventually reverting to old eating habits. Flitting off and on the clean eating path will not change eating habits.

What caused the fall?
The first and most important thing to establish is what caused your temptation. What triggered a fall back to your old eating habits? Was it an emotional event or perhaps an activity that triggered a certain way of eating?

Emotional eating
Perhaps an event or even a conversation has triggered an emotional memory or life shock. Or maybe a stressful situation is causing you to take comfort in food. Loneliness, sadness or anxiety can all be emotional eating triggers but so can happiness or a celebration. We celebrate or reward our successes with food or drink (or both).

Mindless Eating
MIndless eating literally means eating without being aware of it. Consider parts of the day or events when you eat without knowing it. Perhaps you pick at food whilst preparing

meals for your children or nibble through biscuits when stuck in a particularly dull meeting. Phone calls, TV watching or driving are often times for mindless eating.

Habitual eating

This is where you have popcorn because you are at the cinema, or you always have the same coffee on your way to work (you can't survive without it). Or perhaps you can't leave a meal without a sweet treat to finish off. Some habitual eating is also mindless.

Once you've identified what caused your change in eating behaviour (let's call it a binge) be aware of it and move on. Sounds simple doesn't it! But the important point to recognise is that you need to become conscious that this has happened. Recognise the trigger and the reaction rather than allowing it to evolve into negative mind talk which you never acknowledge.

Let's take a simple example:
You've been detoxing for a fortnight. You've lost some weight and you have lots more energy. People have been noticing. So you decide to get yourself a new pair of jeans for a night out. You aren't keen on shopping since things rarely fit but given your weight loss you're feeling positive. You go into one shop and try on some new jeans, perhaps a little more fitted than your usual 'safe' choice but in the changing room the lighting makes the skin on your legs look dimpled and the jeans look dreadful. They leave a roll hanging out of the top and that's before you've managed to do them up.

Does any of this sound familiar?

How do you react?

A: You feel fat. You feel like your good intentions have been a complete waste of time. You tell yourself, 'you will never look good in jeans,' or perhaps, 'you are completely deluded imagining that you might actually look good.' You return the jeans. Put on your 'fat' trousers. Plod out of the shop (not before looking enviously at all the other 'thin' people in the shop) and dive into the nearest chocolate bar, milkshake or chip packet. What's the point anyway?

B: You decide that the jeans you picked up are probably the wrong size, the wrong style or a bad cut and that the lighting in the shop is cheap and unflattering. You'll try somewhere else instead.

How you react is up to you

Whether or not the above scenario is familiar, there are so many different ways of viewing the situation. The jeans don't fit. Fact. But how you react to that fact is up to you. And if you are prone to negative mind chatter, it's possible that a single, misinterpreted situation could cause a massive fall off the detox wagon.

Self-sabotage is only one option

It could be getting on the scales, getting into your gym kit or seeing yourself in a less than flattering mirror. You can't avoid all 'potential' situations. There could be a massive life shock, like an illness in the family or an issue at work but self-sabotage is only one option. It is possible to change the way you react to a situation or setback.

Falling off the wagon doesn't mean it's gone wrong. Yes, it's a setback but treat it as such then move on from the negative thought patterns and behaviour. Turning to food for comfort is just another way of beating yourself up.

How to stay on the wagon?

Be present
If you are always aware of what you are eating, you are less likely to mindlessly pick.

Plan and prepare ahead
If you have planned your food for the day and/or the week, you know what you will be eating. There's no hunger emergency and there's less room for temptation.

Years ago it was mainly body builders who prepared their food for the day ahead in little plastic pots and containers. These days it's much more common (and a bit trendy too). Literally prepare everything you are going to eat in the morning (or the night before) and package it up. That way you know exactly what you are going to eat. You could have something bubbling away in the slow cooker for that 30 minute kids' teatime window or perhaps a salad, layered up in a jar ready to tip onto a plate for your lunch. There are loads of ideas in the book and on my social media pages. You can dip in and choose what works best for you but always ALWAYS plan ahead.

Be accountable
If you are going solo on this it's always going to be tough. Consider a sponsor (a partner or friend who's going to do this with you) or join one of the social media groups I have set up. We have a social media check in every day. You can discuss temptations and set backs as well as the successes of others. It's a great way to stay on track and really succeed.

Affirmations

When it comes to your mindset and your readiness to take on a new challenge, you can't expect to have the same motivation in two weeks as you have today. I mentioned at the start of this book that there's a certain excitement in starting a new diet. It's fun and different. It feels really positive (and slightly smug). But what happens when the same old negativity kicks in? This time I'd like for you to stay positive and on track, rather than slipping back into old habits.

So we've got our lists and we've got our goals. Every day our list includes something that's taking us towards our goals. But what is going to keep us motivated to stay on track?

This is where affirmations come in. Have you tried them before? Affirmations are little statements and sentences that you can refer to or say to yourself when you feel a bit low. They'll help you to stay on track.

When challenges strike it can be easy to get lost in a pity party
We sometimes feel it's not our fault or the world is ganging up against us. And, if you use food as a comfort, the chances are when you have a little pity party, you could feel tempted to indulge in a few 'off plan' treats because it's not really your fault.

We always have a choice in how we feel. No matter how tired, how wronged, how angry or how upset you are, you can always choose to feel positive. I'm not saying it's easy but it's better than having no plans when you feel like this.

Build your toolbox of affirmations

I'd love for you to find affirmations that work for you. From friends or your team who are joining you on *Kick Start Fat Loss*. From the internet or social media. From books that you love. Find them and write them everywhere. On post its. In your purse. On your phone home screen. On your fridge door. Stick them EVERYWHERE.

Here are some that I love, from real women, to get you started:

"Yesterday ended last night. Today is a brand new day and it's mine." [Vivienne Caron Lee]

"Today I choose to only eat healthy nutritious food." [Rachel Holmes]

"Today I unchain myself from all I hate, to set myself free." [Mairi Taylor]

"Today I only make healthy food choices that serve me and my family well." [Mairi Taylor]

"I am charge of how I feel - and today I feel happiness." [Rachel Holmes]

"I don't work hard because I hate my body. I work hard because I love my body." [Rachel Holmes]

"Today I elevate my health, fitness and nutrition." [Rachel Holmes]

"Today I choose to exercise to feel good and positive." [Rachel Holmes]

JoJo Reilly

JoJo Reilly from Drogheda County Louth (Ireland) was fed up of feeling uncomfortable in her own skin. The 39-year-old sales assistant recently lost three stone in three months with *Kick Start Fat Loss* and has swapped feeling uncomfortable for being unstoppable. Here's JoJo's story:

Both weight gain and an expanding waistline meant that leggings and tracksuits had become a wardrobe staple for me. At 39 I was feeling both the physical and emotional restraints from being overweight.

Walking was a chore and often left me feeling tired and out of breath. My diet was rubbish and I did no exercise.

I had constant fatigue and no confidence.

I dreaded socialising and trying on clothes would regularly leave me in floods of tears.
One day I was a passenger in a car, sitting in the front seat and I physically couldn't cross my legs without using my hands to help – I knew then something needed to change.

That change came on 6th January 2015. Weighing in at 12 stone I joined Kick Start Fat Loss run by franchisee Laura Armada Buch. Kick Start Fat Loss is a plan that champions a healthy lifestyle and focuses on real foods which are unprocessed, fresh, seasonal and nutrient dense.

Before Kick Start Fat Loss my daily food intake went something like this: Nothing for breakfast; a chicken sandwich, crisps and chocolate for lunch; and a burger, chips and two litre bottle of coke for dinner.

I now enjoy cooking and eating foods like scrambled eggs with spinach for breakfast, omelettes, fish or meat with broccoli for lunch and chicken stir fry or chilli and vegetables for dinner. The daily two litre bottle of coke has been replaced with water and green tea.

I now plan my meals in advance and have also started going to bed earlier – both of which help keep me on track, plus I'm sleeping so much better.

Within a week of starting Kick Start Fat Loss my energy returned. I felt physically and mentally stronger thanks to the nutritious food I was eating. My diet didn't rely on calorie counting, weighing food or any other methods of restriction. Instead, thanks to Kick Start Fat Loss I began to understand more about the nutritional value and benefits of food.

In three months I had lost three stone. It changed my life. No more sitting on the sofa mindlessly eating. No more emotional binges. No more dieting!

I was exercising too and loving it. The fitness I'd been introduced to by Kick Start Fat Loss boosted my fat loss and also my self- esteem. I now train regularly in Pole fitness, Hot Yoga and HIIT classes – all run by my Kick Start Fat Loss coach Laura Armada Buch.

Shopping for clothes is now a positive experience and socialising with friends and family is fun again. I also used to have pains in my hands, which have now completely gone. I'm sure this is due to changing my diet and giving up fizzy drinks.

Here are my top weight loss and healthy living tips:
- *Plan your meals in advance*
- *Keep a food diary*
- *Take before and after pictures*
- *Join Kick Start Fat Loss and use the ongoing support from both your coach and online forums*
- *Try a different recipe each week*

Remember this is for you and you deserve the best so take it a day at a time, keep that goal in mind and then smash it!

The Kitchen Detox challenge

So far *Kick Start Fat Loss* L has been all about the research and making your mind up. I've got an activity challenge for you now. That means now. Or, if you're reading this in transit, when you get home. Or perhaps make one of your five thing to do today this challenge.

The kitchen detox challenge
This is going to prepare you for your 28 day 'clean eating' detox.

1. Clear out the fridge, pantry, freezer and kitchen of anything likely to cause you to ruin the plan.

2. Dump processed food, packaged, microwave dinners, frozen foods, ready meals – anything packaged, and containing E numbers.

3. Give away all bread, biscuits, cakes and breakfast cereals. Wheat and gluten, for many people, are simply indigestible or place a large stress on the digestive system.

4. Throw out dairy – milk, butter and cheese.

5. Give away all your alcohol (or give it to someone for safe keeping) - that includes wine and spritzers. Alcohol is a toxin your body has to work hard to remove from your system, placing stress on the liver, kidneys and adrenal glands.

6. Remove fizzy drinks, that includes fizzy water.

7. Get rid of all sugar. All forms create an insulin response. The simpler the makeup of the sugar, the more rapid and aggressive the insulin response.

8. No chocolate, sweets or confectionary.

HELP!

What if you have a family or a partner who isn't dieting with you? That's going to be tough. Either get them to come on it with you or they will have to help you so don't get weak and fall into eating any of the foods on the toxic list. You will have to be extra tough if this applies to you.

Kick Start Fat Loss 28 day 'clean eating' detox Shopping List

The beauty of this plan is that you design your own meals. I've provided a complete list of foods and drinks for you to choose from. All your meals need to come from this list and nowhere else. It should make shopping easy and meal planning more creative.

Clean eating plan
This is a clean eating plan. It's designed to get rid of all processed foods. Grass fed beef, organic eggs, and meat are much better quality than standard varieties. Organic animals have been fed with good quality feed, this improves the quality of the meat you are going to consume.

This is also a gluten and dairy free eating plan.

Basic shopping list
This is not exhaustive and there will be additions as we go along.

Protein
- Beef
- Chicken
- Duck
- Turkey
- Lamb
- Liver
- Kidney
- Veal
- Bacon (very lean)
- Shellfish (Shrimp, Crab, Lobster)
- Salmon
- Cod
- Plaice
- Halibut/turbot
- Hake
- Bream
- Prawns
- Rainbow trout
- Haddock
- Mackerel
- Sea bass
- Fresh tuna (not tinned)
- Eggs

If you are able to afford organic, then choose organic and local produce wherever possible.

Ensure vegetables are fresh, washed and peeled before you eat them.

Steam, grill, poach and lightly fry fish and meat.

Carbohydrates

Eat as many green vegetables as you can with every meal.
Vegetables to eat freely include:
- Spinach
- Courgette
- Cucumber
- Broccoli
- Rocket
- Aubergine
- Squash
- All leafy greens
- Tomatoes
- Onion
- Kale
- Cabbage
- Celery
- Mushrooms
- Peas
- Green peppers
- Green beans
- Purple sprouting broccoli
- Broad beans
- Cauliflower
- Avocado

Fats

- Use coconut oil freely to cook with.
- Flavour your food with olive oil (don't cook with it as it doesn't react well to high temperatures).

Nuts

If you struggle to eat just a few nuts at a time, then go easy on them! We call these domino foods since once you have a few, you are compelled to eat the whole lot.
- Almonds
- Macadamia Nuts

Extras on Carb Days

Keep away from high sugar fruits. Only eat berries/bananas on carb days or after training.
- Brown rice
- Sweet potato
- Fruit
- Quinoa

Drink

- Water (minimum 3 litres per day)
- Fruit teas
- Liquorice
- Tulsi tea

The *Kick Start Fat Loss* Plan

Kick Start Fat Loss Key Basics

- Eat three meals per day.
- No snacking between meals.
- Ensure you eat plenty at every meal and fill up on vegetables.
- Perform a daily 10-minute HIIT Workout from the Kickstartfatloss.net website before breakfast.
- Aim to drink 2-3 litres of bottled water daily.
- Drink fruit teas, especially liquorice and tulsi tea.
- Plan your meals in advance and use your slow cooker.
- Only choose foods from the shopping list to make up your meals.

Kick Start Fat Loss Meal Planner

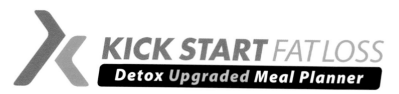

KICK START *FAT LOSS*
Detox Upgraded Meal Planner

DAY 1	DAY 2	DAY 3	DAY 4	DAY 5	DAY 6	DAY 7
BREAKFAST	**BREAKFAST**	**BREAKFAST**	**BREAKFAST**	**BREAKFAST**	**BREAKFAST**	**BREAKFAST**
Stir Fry optional Meat /Prawns	Frittata-Eggs Vegetables	Omelette Scrambled Eggs	Meat choice with Vegetables	Stir Fry Vegetables	Fish Choice with Vegetables	Organic Bacon Eggs with Vegetables
1 - 2 TBSP Coconut Oil	1 - 2 TBSP Coconut Oil	1 - 2 TBSP Coconut Oil	1 - 2 TBSP Coconut Oil	1 - 2 TBSP Coconut Oil	1 - 2 TBSP Coconut Oil	1 - 2 TBSP Coconut Oil
1 TBSP Organic Butter / Ghee	Olive Oil	1 TBSP Organic Butter / Ghee	Olive Oil	1 TBSP Organic Butter / Ghee	Olive Oil	1 TBSP Organic Butter / Ghee

Eat meal 1 when you are ready to eat it doesn't have to first thing in the morning · No snacking between meals · Eat till you feel full full not stuffed · Really chew your food well so the stomach doesn't have to do all of the work · If you are allergic to diary or butter go for Organic Ghee & Coconut or MCT Oil for Fats

LUNCH	LUNCH	LUNCH	LUNCH	LUNCH	LUNCH	LUNCH
Meat Choice with Green Vegetables	Fish Choice with Green Vegetables	Meat Choice with Green Vegetables	Egg with Meat or Fish Choice with Green vegetables	Meat Choice with Green Vegetables	Fish Choice with Green Vegetables	Egg with Meat or Fish Choice with Green Vegetables
1 x Avocado		Nuts (sml qantity)	1 x Avocado		1 x Avocado	Nuts (sml qantity)
1 TBSP Organic Butter / Ghee + 1 TBSP Coconut Oil	1 TBSP Organic Butter / Ghee + 1 TBSP Coconut Oi	1 TBSP Organic Butter / Ghee + 1 TBSP Coconut Oil	1 TBSP Organic Butter / Ghee + 1 TBSP Coconut Oil	1 TBSP Organic Butter / Ghee + 1 TBSP Coconut Oil	1 TBSP Organic Butter / Ghee + 1 TBSP Coconut Oil	1 TBSP Organic Butter / Ghee + 1 TBSP Coconut Oil

Rotate your meats and fishes (protein choices)

DINNER	DINNER	DINNER	DINNER	DINNER	DINNER	DINNER
Egg with Meat or Fish Choice with Green vegetables	Meat Choice with Green Vegetables	Fish Choice with Green Vegetables	Meat or Fish Choice with Green vegetables	Fish Choice with Green Vegetables	Meat Choice with Green Vegetables	Meat or Fish Choice with Green Vegetables
1 TBSP Organic Butter / Ghee + 1 TBSP Coconut Oil	1 TBSP Organic Butter / Ghee + 1 TBSP Coconut Oi	1 TBSP Organic Butter / Ghee + 1 TBSP Coconut Oil	1 TBSP Organic Butter / Ghee + 1 TBSP Coconut Oil	1 TBSP Organic Butter / Ghee + 1 TBSP Coconut Oil	1 TBSP Organic Butter / Ghee + 1 TBSP Coconut Oil	1 TBSP Organic Butter / Ghee + 1 TBSP Coconut Oil

PAR Q

Par Q and Physical Activity Questionnaire

We need to assess that you are healthy and suitable to do the KSFL exercise workouts. If in any doubt, please contact your GP or, if you have any special medical conditions, always check with your doctor before embarking on the KSFL.

1   Has your doctor ever said you have a heart condition and that you should only do physical activity recommended by a doctor?
2   Do you feel pain in your chest when you do physical activity?
3   In the past month, have you had a chest pain when you were not doing physical activity?
4   Do you suffer from asthma - if so, do you use inhalers?
5   Are you diabetic?
6   Do you have a bone or joint problem (e.g. back, knee or hip) that could be made worse by a change in your physical activity?
7   Are you pregnant or have you been pregnant in the last 6 months?
8   Are you currently taking any medication? If yes, what and for what reason?
9   Do you suffer from regular back pain or have you had any back injury?
10 Do you know of any other reason why you shouldn't exercise?

'I have read, understood and accurately completed this questionnaire. I confirm that I am voluntarily engaging in an acceptable level of exercise, and my participation involves a risk of injury.'

Client Name ....

Signature .... Date .... DOB ....

Telephone .... Email ....

KSFL Leader Name ....

Signature .... Date ....

Breakfast recipe ideas

These are so quick and easy, and are *Kick Start Fat Loss* staples.

Stir fries are also great for breakfasts.

Boiled Eggs 'Hollandaise'

Boil your egg and cut into quarters.
Top with a knob of grass fed butter.
Chop avocado and place on top.

Frittata

In a frying pan over medium heat lightly fry courgettes, broccoli and peppers in coconut oil.
Crack 3 eggs into a bowl and whisk.
Pour the eggs into the pan.
Allow to cook for 5 minutes then flip over and cook for a further 5 minutes or until golden brown on each side.

Ultimate Green Juice

Juice the following ingredients:
1 bunch celery
4-5 kale leaves
1 green apple
1 handful parsley
1 lime
1 lemon
1 inch fresh ginger

Lunch recipe ideas

The key is planning ahead. Try cooking and packing your lunch the night before.

Vegetable Soup

Put a teaspoon of coconut oil into a saucepan.
Chop and sweat off 1 carrot, 2 florets of broccoli, 1 onion, a handful of cabbage and 1 stick of celery.
Pour in 500ml of vegetable stock and allow to simmer for 10 minutes.
Season to taste.
Blend with a hand blender.

Smoked Salmon Asparagus

Boil 1 egg and set aside.
Lightly fry your asparagus in melted coconut oil and season with salt and pepper.
Roll your smoked salmon slices with a rolling pin so they are nice and thin.
Remove the asparagus and wrap the salmon around the spears.
Dunk away!

Turkey Salad

Spread coconut oil onto 1 turkey breast and grill.
Chop 1 handful lettuce, 1/4 cucumber, 4 cherry tomatoes and 1 avocado.
Place your salad in a bowl and drizzle with extra virgin olive oil.
Once the turkey is cooked, slice and place on top of your salad.
Season to taste.

Dinner recipe ideas

Invest in a slow cooker since it's the best way to maintain all of the goodness in your food and it is easy.

Steak, Eggs and Tomato

Grill 1 steak per person.
Fry 2 eggs in coconut oil and set aside.
Grill 4 tomatoes in the same pan.
Plate up all together and season to taste.

Vegetable Stew

Heat a teaspoon of coconut oil large, heavy-based pan.
Add 1 onion and cook gently for 5 –10 minutes until softened.
Add 3 cloves chopped garlic, dried thyme, 3 carrots, 2 sticks of celery and 2 peppers and cook for 5 minutes.
Add 800g peeled cherry tomatoes, 250ml vegetable stock and fresh thyme and cook for 20 - 25 minutes.
Take out the thyme sprigs.
Stir in 250g cooked lentils and bring back to a simmer.

Fish and Cauliflower Rice

Place the following ingredients in tin foil on a baking tray:
2 pieces of white fish, squeeze over 1 lemon, sprinkle a little salt and pepper, place 6 cherry tomatoes around the fish and fold the foil over to create a package.
Cook in the oven at 180c for 25 minutes.
Check it is cooked and serve with the cauliflower rice.

For the cauliflower rice:
Heat a frying pan and add a teaspoon of coconut oil.
Grate in cauliflower.

The *Kick Start Fat Loss* Fit Test

Before you embark on any fitness programme, we need to establish exactly from where you are starting.

We can then measure your exact progress over the 28 days.

10 exercises
Here are the 10 exercises you need to perform as a workout on day one of your *Kick Start Fat Loss*. You will then perform the fit test every seven days and record your scores. There is an online video with all of the exercises demonstrated for your information.

Do each exercise for 40 seconds, rest for 20 seconds and record your scores below.

Ensure you warm up before you start (see the next chapter for ideas). We can then track you progress and fitness levels.

1. Power Squat
2. Split Lunge
3. Tricep Dips
4. V Sit
5. Burpee
6. Press Up
7. Hill Climber
8. Corkscrew Burpee
9. Tuck Jumps
10. High Knee Runs

Home Workout Diary

Always perform a five minute warm up before your workout. This could include walking, jogging, skipping, in fact, any activity that will elevate your heart rate before the 10-minute HIIT workout.

Details of your daily home workouts will be emailed to you when you have registered your details on www.KickStartFatLoss.net

Additional workouts can also be found on the private *Kick Start Fat Loss* Facebook page.

Cool down and perform the stretches taught to you in the LIVE class.

Food and Mood Diary

Buy a new notebook and write down everything you have eaten and drunk through the day.

Also, note how the food made you feel and a rough portion size. This will help us tweak your diet as you go.

You can use this page for now if you don't have a note book to hand.

Scales are for fish

Although it's very tempting to weigh yourself daily, please try not to.

The reasons are multiple, some people will lose more weight at the beginning of this program and others will lose more weight towards the end.

The *Kick Start Fat Loss* programme regulates your hormones, therefore your weight could swing up or down as much as three or four pounds every day.

Focus on your inch loss
Your measurements are more important than what you see on the scales, which is why I focus on your inch loss and how you look from week to week with your photos.

In addition, it can be heartbreaking for some people who jump on the scales after seven or 14 days and see they haven't lost as much weight as other people. We all lose weight at different speeds. Your measurements and photos are 90% more important than what the scales say.

We only use the scales as a guide. Once a week on our results day.

It is tempting to continually jump on the scales several times a day but it's really not helpful and is only part of your *Kick Start Fat Loss* results.

Remember - scales are for fish!

Photos and measurements

The Camera Never Lies
With any eating plan, weeks three and four are where your body shape really starts to change and adapt, which is why this plan is 28 days.

You may find that your weight loss stabilises, so it's really all about your inch loss and shape change, especially with the workouts I have planned for you.

Photos are VITAL to track your success
This is why photos are so important. In fact, before and after photos are not just important but VITAL to track your success, yet many people don't want to take them as they make them feel uncomfortable.

BUT YOU MUST.

Why?

The camera never lies.
We can compare photos along the way and at the end to measure progress.

During times of 'I can't do this' we can compare our before photo to our most recent pictures and think 'look how far I have come.'

So please take the following photographs:
• From the front
• From the side
• From the back

Please post in the group. It keeps us all on track and accountable.

Measurements
Please take the following measurements today:
• Chest
• Waist
• Hips
• Both thighs
• Both arms

Then add all of the measurements together for your total inches (TI).

Please keep your pictures on your phone or on your home PC. You can also post your details in the Facebook group. Or join a *Kick Start Fat Loss* group. You don't have to go in person (although evidence shows that those who do are more successful in the long run).

Life after the *Kick Start Fat Loss* detox

Congratulations beautiful lady.

You have made it to the end of the best detox out there.

Well done.

You have reached the end of the biggest and toughest stage of your *Kick Start Fat Loss* journey.

How does it feel?

I really hope, that like so many of my *Kick Start Fat Loss* army, you are feeling invincible.

I've been working in the fitness industry for nearly thirty years now and I can't tell you how much I love the amazing results that my team are getting.

I am buzzing with the excitement of it all.

So where do you go from here?

I get women asking me this all the time. They've got to the end of the detox. They've made massive changes to the way they eat, drink, exercise and think. And they want to find a way to incorporate the *Kick Start Fat Loss* principles into their lifestyle, for good.

They want to feel this invincible, for good.

And I love this question. This is what I want for you.

Binge with caution

I'm going to start with a few words of caution.

Now is not the time to celebrate with a binge. It will just make you feel horrible.

I know that after detoxing, it can be tempting to party. Hard. And by party I mean indulge in a few drinks and sugary treats.

But believe me, from ladies I know who have done this, you will just feel awful for days. It's a recipe for the hangover to beat all hangovers.

You've been through a process of detoxing your body and training your body, especially your liver to be an efficient energy machine. It's forgotten about processing alcohol.

Throughout the detox we've covered so much of the science and research behind what makes a truly healthy diet, for life. So fortunately, in terms of maintaining the changes you've made to your lifestyle, you are already armed with so much knowledge and understanding that you already have a lot of the answers.

But just in case you need a little encouragement, here are some pointers for maintaining the *Kick Start Fat Loss* lifestyle:

Kick Start Fat Loss Maintenance

- Be a Diet Detective. Seek out those nasties in processed foods, whatever the marketing label says.
- Just walk past all those processed foods. They need you more than you need them.
- If you have a cheat meal (and cheat meals are okay) recognise that you've had a cheat meal, even plan it and then move on.
- Don't turn your cheat meal into a cheat graze, day, or week!
- Live a guilt free life. You can eat what you want. But now you know how your body will react to it.
- You can still be a foodie and eat the *Kick Start Fat Loss* way. In fact I really hope that you're even more of a foodie now than when you started reading the book.
- Share your journey with your friends. Encourage everyone who needs a little push in the right direction. Be their inspiration.

Eating out tips

What about nights or meals out?

There's no reason you can't still enjoy meals out. You may want to classify them as cheat meals but there are ways to ensure you stick with the main *Kick Start Fat Loss* principles whilst you dine out.

Choose meat/fish and vegetables and skip the potatoes or heavy carbohydrate based dishes.

And for all budding bakers ...

You can still enjoy baking but think about substitutes for refined sugar and flour. Get creative. There are loads of brilliant baking recipes in my *Kick Start Fat Loss* cook book.

The next steps on your *Kick Start Fat Loss* journey

So you've done the detox and you're on a high. Congratulations.

This isn't the end though, this is just the beginning.

Now that you've begun to understand how to look after your body I hope that you'll stay with us on the journey.

Nutritional science is constantly evolving, along with exercise science. Scientists are beginning to understand what we need to eat to minimise our risk of disease, just by looking at our DNA.

Don't forget that after all your success, your friends might want to know your secret. Don't be afraid to share it. In fact shout it.

How do you feel?

You are armed with some cracking information to make some radical changes.

Remember ... dependent on your personality type, you might be an all or nothing type (like me) someone who says 'right I'm on this, clean the pantry, call the organic farm, get onto the grass fed butcher, ditch the cereal. I'm all over this 10000%' - or you might think 'eeekkkk, I would rather do this in smaller steps, I'll change my breakfast first, then I'll settle into that, then I'll look at my sugar and alcohol'. Both approaches are PERFECT.

Perfect for you as an individual.

You will both still get there.

Set yourself up for success and take the approach that is right for your personality.

Overhauling your lifestyle takes time and perseverance, just keep moving in the right direction.

If you need help, support and motivation then find me on social media.

I LOVE to hear from you and I'm constantly writing articles, making vlogs and audios with all the very latest *Kick Start Fat Loss* tips and updates so tune in and get involved.

Join the revolution!

Tweet me @RachelHolmes #KSFLREV

Like KSFL on Facebook www.Facebook.com/KickStartFatLoss

Follow me on Instagram @RachelLHolmes